Gallstones - Review and Recent Progress

Edited by Qiang Yan and Huaping Shen

Published in London, United Kingdom

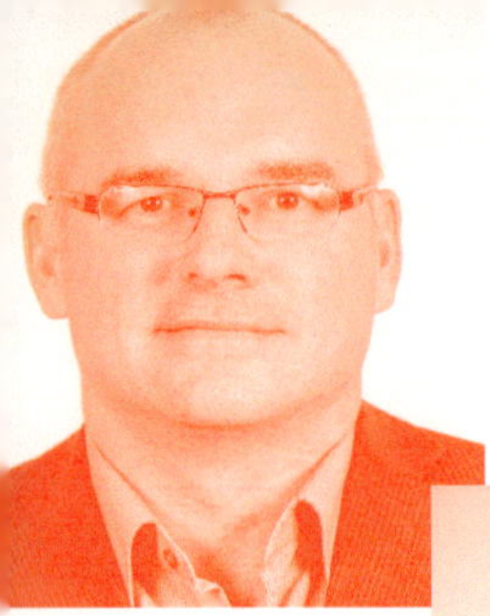
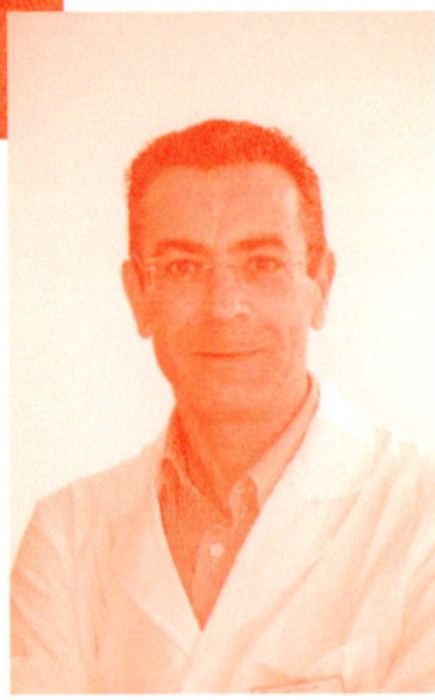
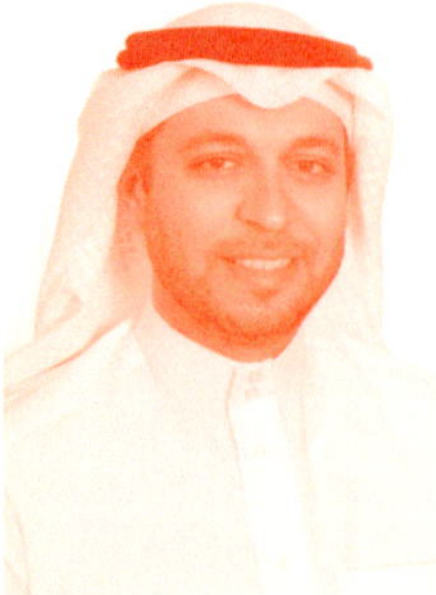
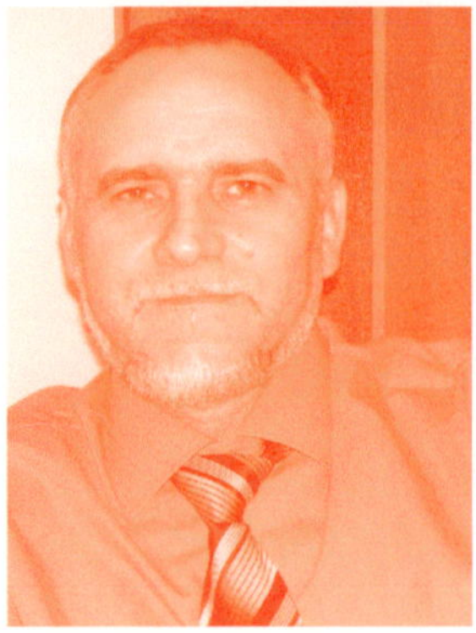
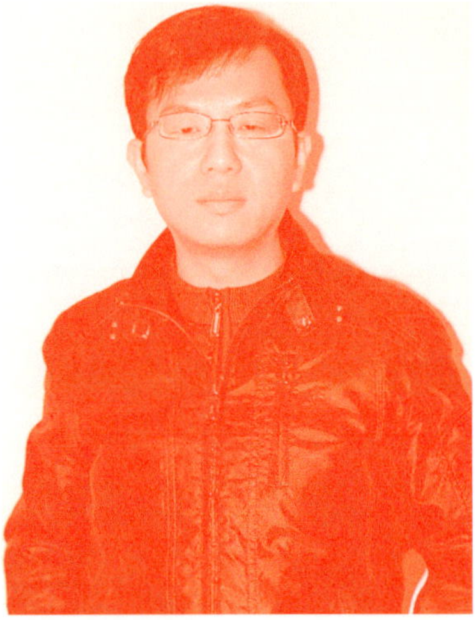
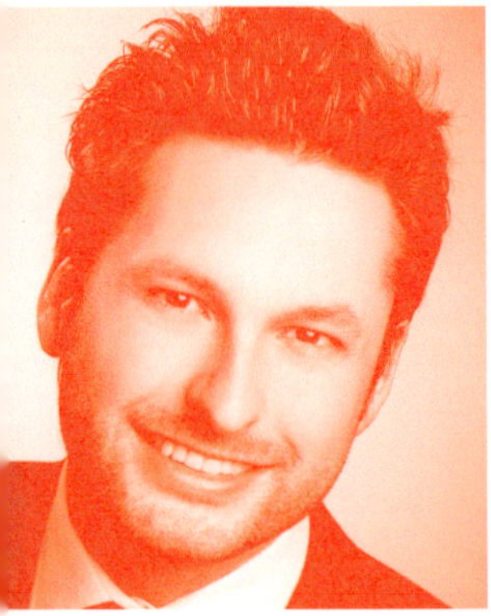
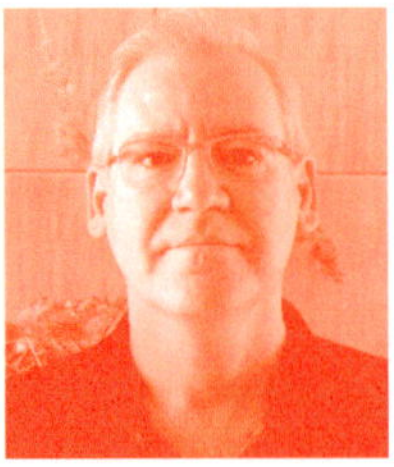

IntechOpen

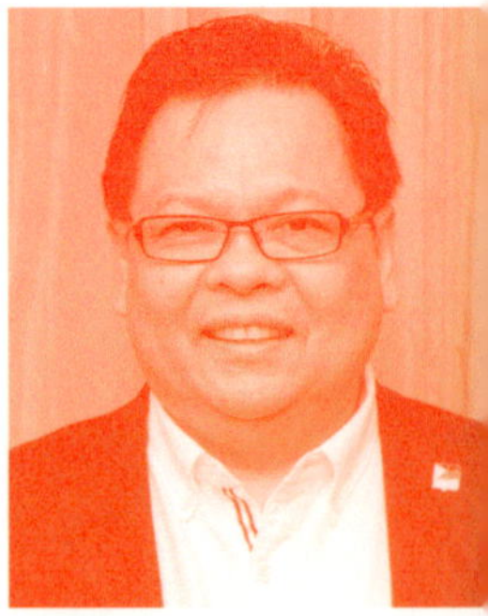
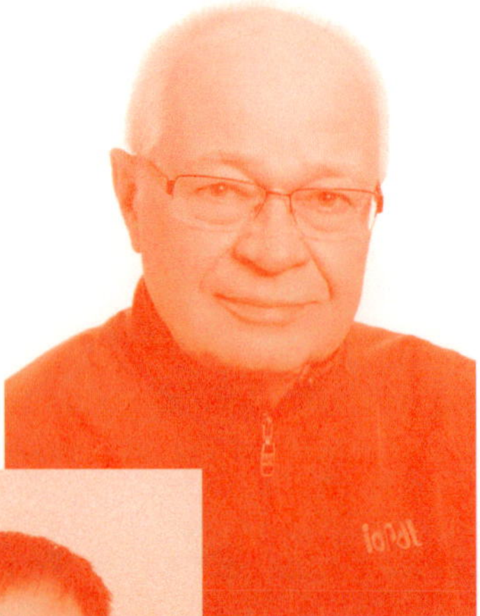
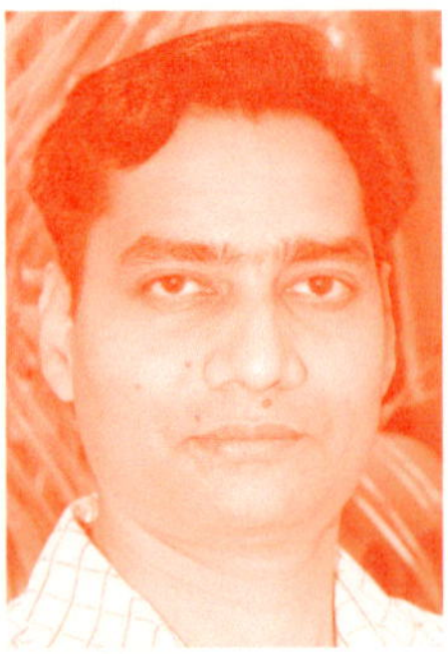
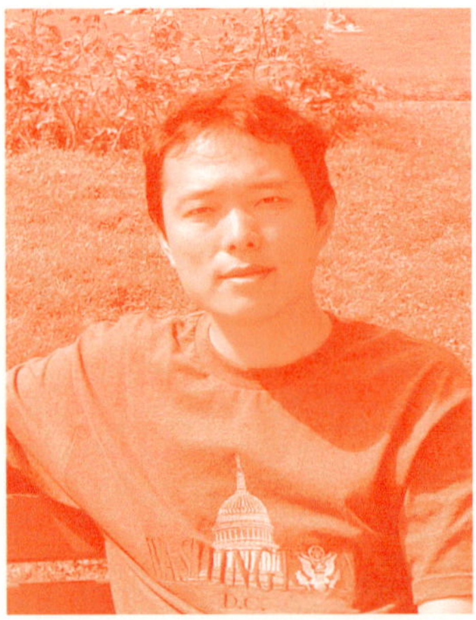
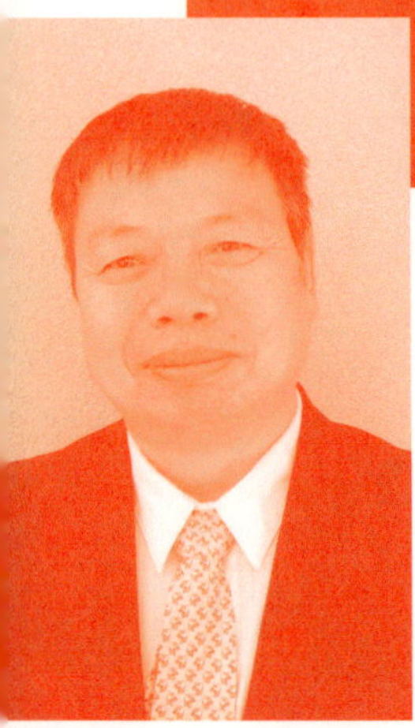
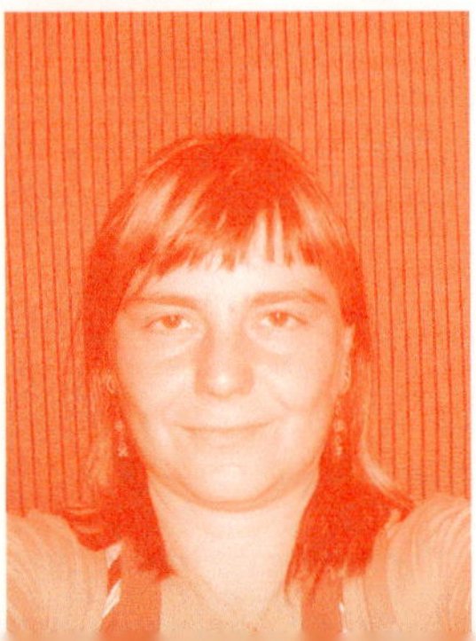

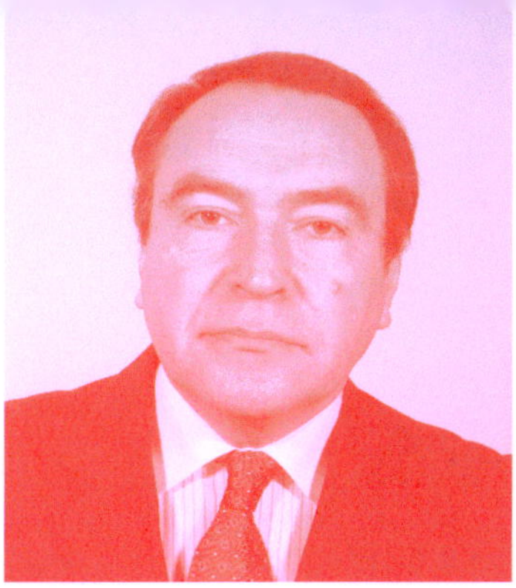
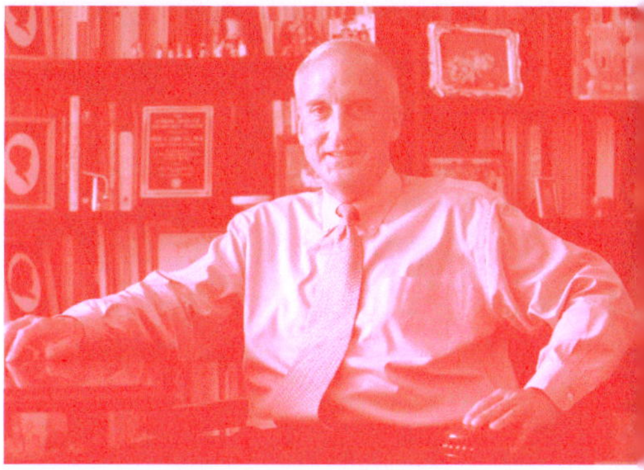
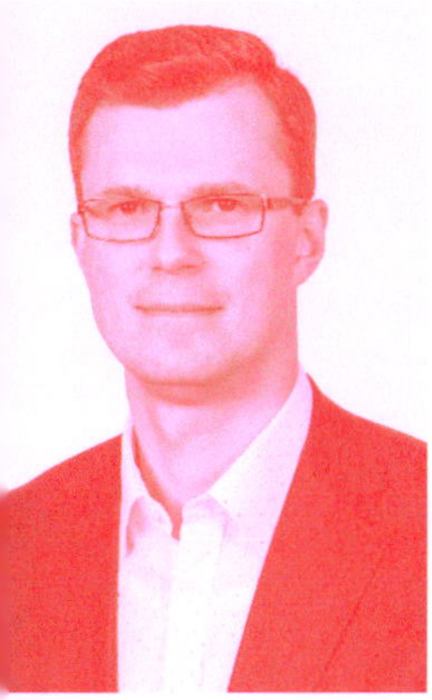
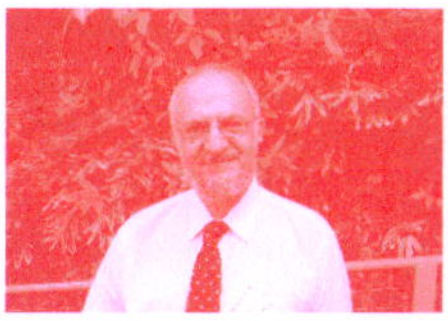
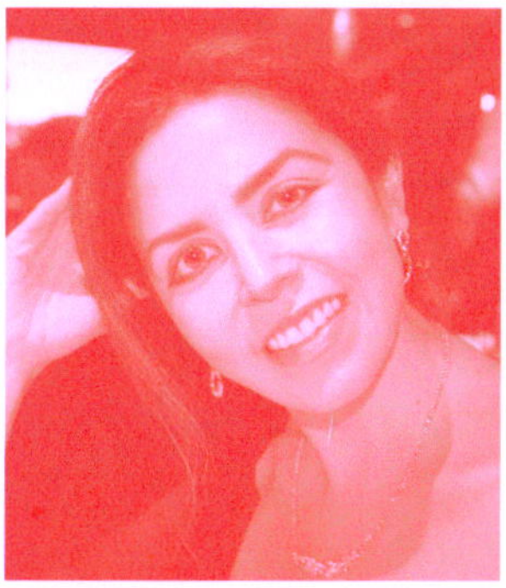

Supporting open minds since 2005

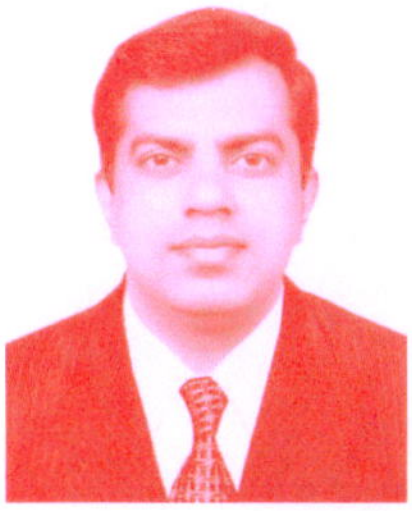
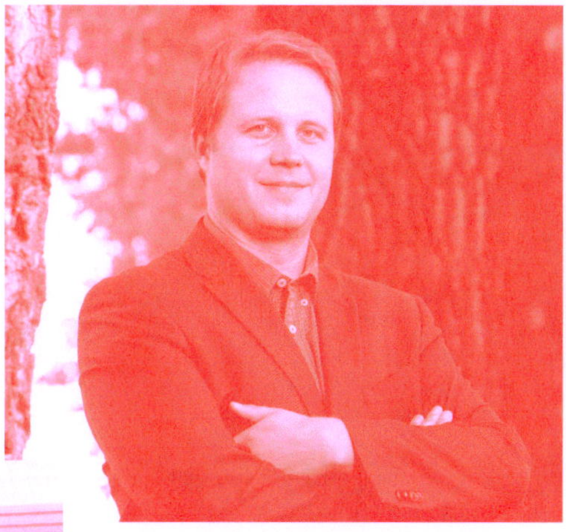
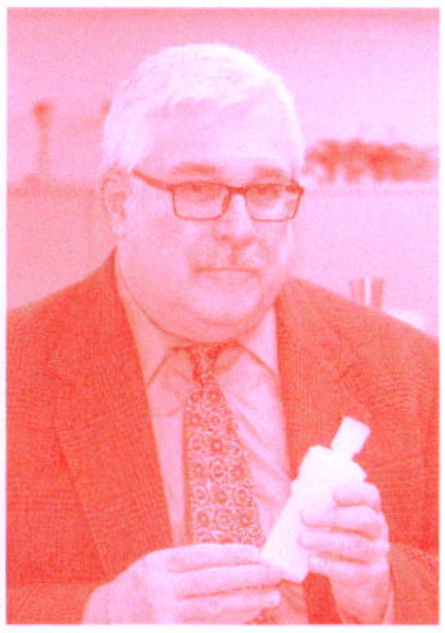
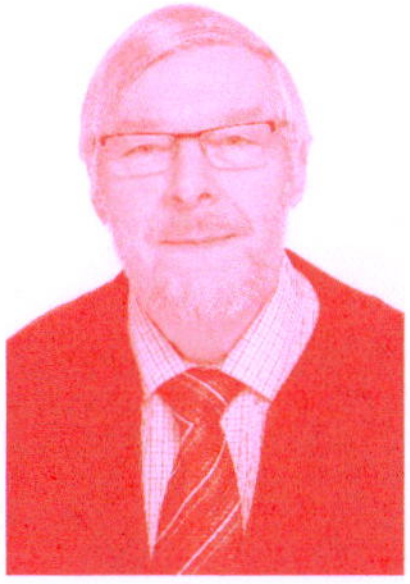
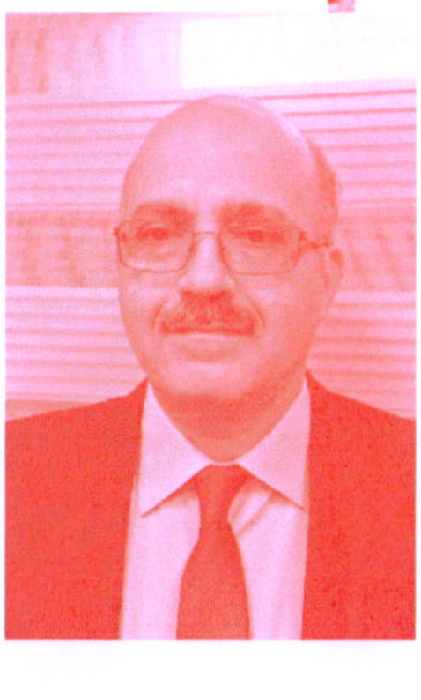
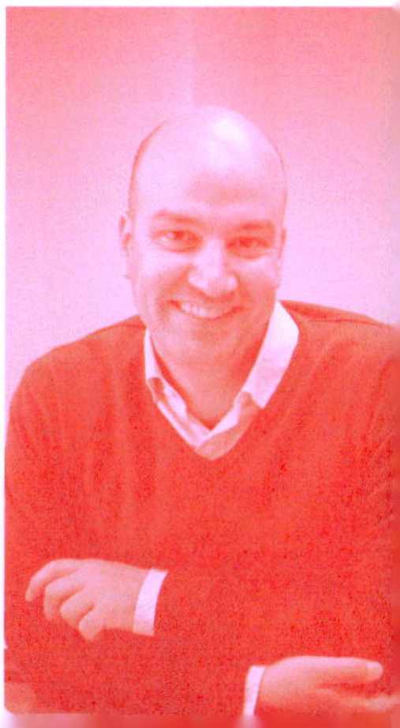
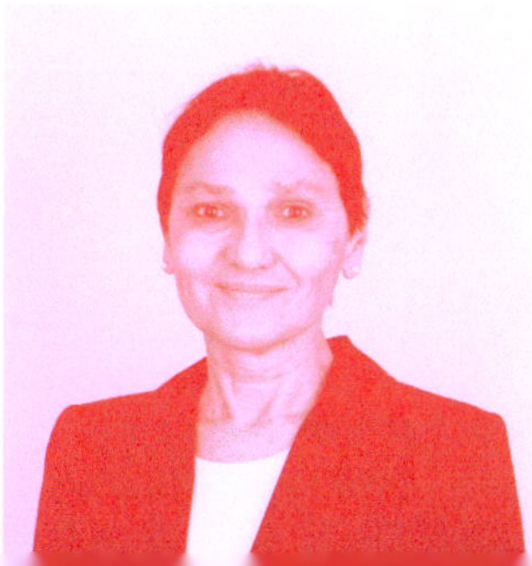

Gallstones - Review and Recent Progress
http://dx.doi.org/10.5772/intechopen.94688
Edited by Qiang Yan and Huaping Shen

Contributors
Giovanni Petracca, Fabrizio Silvaggio, Francesco Zappia, Giuseppe Maccarone, Mariano Mazzeo, Francesco Mio, Irshad Ahmad Kumar, Ferkhand Mohi Ud Din, Ashiq Hussain Raina, Mela Ram Attri, Aakarshit Attri, Nida Mirza Shaikh, Hirotaka Okamoto, Peter Dubovan, Miroslav Tomáš, Ramadan Aziri, Hema Prakash Kumari Pilli, Vijayalakshmi Payala, Cosmas Rinaldi A Rinaldi A. Lesmana, Laurentius A. Lesmana, Mileto Ivana, Plutino Francesco, Posterino Antonietta, Danilo Cafaro

First published in London, United Kingdom, 2022 by IntechOpen
IntechOpen is the global imprint of INTECHOPEN LIMITED, registered in England and Wales, registration number: 11086078, 5 Princes Gate Court, London, SW7 2QJ, United Kingdom
Printed in Croatia

British Library Cataloguing-in-Publication Data
A catalogue record for this book is available from the British Library

Additional hard and PDF copies can be obtained from orders@intechopen.com

Gallstones - Review and Recent Progress
Edited by Qiang Yan and Huaping Shen
p. cm.
Print ISBN 978-1-83880-675-0
Online ISBN 978-1-83880-676-7
eBook (PDF) ISBN 978-1-83880-677-4

For EU product safety concerns:
IN TECH d.o.o., Prolaz Marije Krucifikse Kozulić 3, 51000 Rijeka, Croatia, info@intechopen.com or visit our website at intechopen.com.

Meet the editors

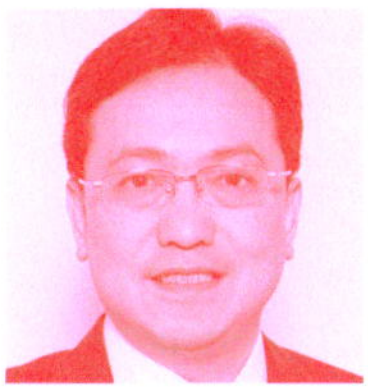

Qiang Yan, MD, is a master's supervisor, adjunct professor, and *Fellow of the American College of Surgeons* (FACS). He is the chairman of the Department of General Surgery and the director of the Department of Hepatopancreatic and Biliary Surgery and Department of Surgery Teaching and Research, Zhejiang University Huzhou Hospital. Dr. Yan is a member of the Committees of Biliary Surgeons, Department of Surgeons and Hepatobiliary Minimal of Non-invasive Surgery, Chinese Medical Doctor Association, and many other academic associations. He is also a special member of the editorial committees of the *Chinese Journal of General Surgery*, *Liver Cancer*, and *Chinese Journal of Clinicians*. He is a participant in the High-Level Talents of Zhejiang Medicine and Zhejiang Province 151 Talents. Dr. Yan completed advanced studies in hepatobiliary pancreatic surgery at Stanford University Medical Center, California, and *University Hospital Regensburg, Germany.* He has more than thirty high-quality papers to his credit.

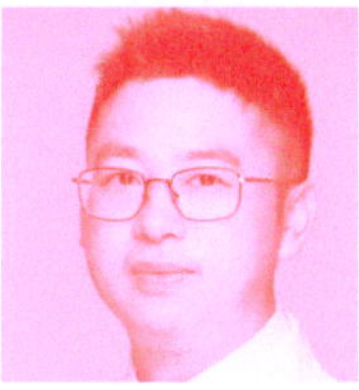

Huaping Shen is an associate chief of the Department of Hepatopancreatic and Biliary (HPB) Surgery, Zhejiang University Huzhou Hospital. He has been engaged in hepatobiliary and pancreatic surgery for 10 years and is an expert in diagnosis and treatment of hepatobiliary and pancreatic diseases. Dr. Shen has ten medical papers to his credit and has participated in seven research projects.

Contents

Preface

Recently, the prevalence of gallstones has increased, and the pattern of gallstones has changed. Most gallstones are found in the gallbladder, but they sometimes pass through the cystic duct into extrahepatic and/or intrahepatic bile ducts to become bile-duct stones, causing conditions known as choledocholithiasis and hepatolithiasis. Gallstones may cause a series of clinical symptoms such as biliary obstruction, infection, and even malignant transformation. There are also some gallstone patients who never experience symptoms. At present, there is still a lot of discussion about the causes and prevention of gallstones. With the renewal of treatment concepts, treatment strategies such as laparoscopic technology, puncture technology, and endoscopic technology have become the main methods for treating gallstones. However, these methods can also bring about a variety of complications.

This book discusses the epidemiological and pathophysiological characteristics of gallstones, the latest progress in the treatment of different types of gallstones, and the management of complications. It provides clinicians with evidence for clinical decision-making and provides scientists with a comprehensive overview of current developments in this vital area.

Qiang Yan
Department of General Surgery,
Huzhou Central Hospital,
Hu Zhou, China

Huaping Shen
Zhejiang University Huzhou Hospital,
Hu Zhou, China

Chapter 1

Gall Stones in Pediatric Population

Nida Mirza Shaikh

Abstract

Gall stones is a known entity in adults, but are considered uncommon in pediatric population, however in the recent years, mainly with wide spread use of ultrasonography, cholelithiasis in children is being frequently reported. Etiology of gall stones in children is not similar to adults. Pigment stones are the most frequently seen in children with hemolytic disease as the most common cause, however with the increase in obesity in children there is also rise in cholesterol stones. Many other causes like drugs, congenital hepatobiliary malformation and genetic causes are to be kept during evaluation of gall stones. Management of gall stones need a proper and timely work up for the causes of cholelithiasis is necessary in children. Surgical management with laparoscopic cholecystectomy is the treatment of choice in most of the cases however the timing of surgery should be optimized case to case basis.

Keywords: cholelithiasis in children, hemolytic anemia, pseudolithiasis

1. Introduction

Gall stones is a known entity in adults, but are considered uncommon in pediatric population with a prevalence of 0.13% to 0.2% [1] and no clear approach has been defined. However, in the recent years, mainly with wide spread use of ultrasonography, cholelithiasis in children is being frequently reported. Unlike adults the asymptomatic presentation is less likely in children (17–50%) [2, 3]. In children there is no difference in both genders pre pubertal, however there is female predominance after puberty. In some other cases, they are reported in association with clinical symptoms such as cholecystitis and cholangitis [4, 5]. Etiology of gall stones in children is not similar to adults. Many studies have shown haemolytic diseases are the most common causes of cholelithiasis in children [20–30%], followed by other cause like obesity, total parenteral nutrition, ileal disease or resection, congenital hepatobiliary diseases, use of ceftriaxone and idiopathic [6]. Other causes like metabolic syndrome, PFIC (progressive familial intrahepatic cholestasis), choledochal cyst, biliary cirrhosis, prematurity, necrotizing enterocolitis (NEC), Wilson disease, congenital heart diseases, cystic fibrosis, should also be considered.

2. Pathogenesis

Bile is mainly made up of water, bilirubin, cholesterol, bile pigments, and phospholipids. Imbalance in bile constituents [cholesterol, phospholipids, and bile salts] is the main cause of gallstone formation. Gallstone formation starts from the sedimentation of cholesterol, bile pigments, and calcium salts which are insoluble [7]. By composition gallstones are divided into cholesterol gallstones or pigment stones. Unlike adults where mixed cholesterol gallstones are more common in adults, pigment stones are more common in children except adolescent girls.

2.1 Biliary sludge

Biliary sludge is mixture of mucin, calcium bilirubinate and cholesterol crystals, seen with prolonged fasting, sickle-cell disease, total parenteral nutrition, pregnancy and treatment with drugs like ceftriaxone, octreotide etc. [8]. Biliary sludge may resolve spontaneously or on removal of causative agent or may progress to gallstone development. Persistent sludge may give rise to complication like pancreatitis or cholangitis.

2.2 Cholesterol stones

Cholesterol supersaturation of bile with stasis predisposes to cholesterol gallstone formation, increased concentration of cholesterol also elevates the rate of crystallization leading to gallstone formation [9]. The cholesterol content is usually greater than 50%, with minimal calcium content, cholesterol stones are solitary, yellow-white, hard, crystalline, faceted, round, and smooth [10]. These stones are not radiopaque. Formation of cholesterol stones occurs due to hypersecretion of cholesterol, increased mucin production, and decreased gallbladder motility. Cholesterol stones are not commonly seen in children except adolescent girls. The risk factors for cholesterol stone formation in children include obesity, Hispanic ethnicity, family history, female sex (after puberty), and non-alcoholic fatty liver disease.

2.3 Pigment stones

Black pigment stones are formed due to supersaturation of bile with calcium bilirubinate [(to excess bilirubin) and are seen in haemolytic disorders and in association with total parenteral nutrition. These stones are commonly seen with hereditary haemolytic anaemias such as sickle cell disease, hereditary spherocytosis and thalassemia. Pigment stones are also seen with cirrhosis, total parenteral nutrition, ileal disease and ceftriaxone use. Black pigment stones are black to brown in color, hard, shiny, and crystalline, multiple, size of less than 5 mm, composed mainly of bile pigment polymer (40%) followed by calcium carbonate or phosphate, salts, cholesterol and mucin glycoprotein. Persons with Gilbert syndrome, are at increased risk for black pigment gallstones due to increased bilirubin production and a decrease in the bilirubin diphosphate-glucuronosyltransferase activity. Other etiologies for pigmented stones include medications such as ceftriaxone and octreotide. A decrease in the enterohepatic circulation of bile acids (seen with ileal disease or after ileal resection) is another predisposing factor for black stone formation. The mechanism responsible for gallstone formation in this setting is an interruption in the normal enterohepatic circulation of the endogenous bile salt pool [11].

Brown pigment stones are brown to orange in color, soft, greasy, multiple, and smooth composed mainly of calcium bilrubinate [60%] followed by, calcium palmitate, stearate soaps, cholesterol and mucin glycoprotein. Brown pigment stones are distinctly seen in the setting of a bacterial/parasitic infection and biliary stasis. These are also seen in bile duct anomaly and cirrhosis. These are more often seen in the bile ducts than in the gall bladder [12].

2.4 Hemolysis

Cholelithiasis is a well-known complication in pediatric patients with hemolytic anaemias like sickle cell disease, hereditary spherocytosis etc. The prevalence rate of gall stones in sickle cell disease ranges from 30 to 70% which increases progressively with age and is usually not seen before the age of five [13]. The prevalence of pigment gallstones in sickle cell disease is around 10% in children under 10 years of age, which increases to 40% in those aged 10–18 years, and 50% in adults [14–16]. The prevalence of gallstones in hereditary spherocytosis is 10–20% in children, while it raises to 40% in adult population [17, 18]. Incidence of gall stones in thalassemia is low as compared to sickle cell disease [19, 20]. Thalassaemic who also has Gilbert's syndrome genotype shows higher prevalence of gall stones [21, 22]. Whenever a child or adult with sickle cell disease experiences an episode of abdominal pain, cholelithiasis or biliary colic should be considered as differential diagnosis along with vaso-occlusive crisis. In sickle cell disease mutated red blood cells in the oxygenated form do not cause any problems, however in the deoxygenated form, they acquire sickle-like shape due to bond formation between replaced amino acid and globin molecules. This change in shape of red blood cells is reversible by reoxygenation however, changing shape again and again ruptures the cell membrane, which leads to hemolysis [23]. The bilirubin which is produced by hemolysis, further conjugated in the liver and excreted in the intestine as urobilinogen which is further absorbed and excreted multiple times through the enterohepatic circulation of bile.in hemolysis the abundance of urobilinogen in the bile leads to precipitation which may become calcified, which if continuous leads to gall stone formation [24].

2.5 Ceftriaxone-associated biliary pseudolithiasis

Ceftriaxone, is a third-generation cephalosporin, and is commonly used as broad-spectrum antibiotic in children. Gall stones or biliary sludge has been reported as a complication of ceftriaxone treatment since long [25]. The incidence of ceftriaxone induced pseudolithiasis is variable from 15–45%, depending on dose, duration and predisposing host factors [26–30]. Since biliary lithiasis is reversible and disappears on discontinuation of drug it has been termed pseudolithiasis [31]. Ceftriaxone is 40% excreted via bile, as an anion it concentrates in bile easily and readily forms an insoluble salt with calcium [calcium-ceftriaxone] that precipitates in gallbladder [32]. The predisposing risk factors for ceftriaxone induced biliary lithiasis are, high dose (>2 g or >200 mg/kg/day), long-term treatment, hypercalcemia, renal failure, and gallbladder stasis [33]. The mechanism of ceftriaxone induced lithiasis is explained in **Figure 1**. Most cases of ceftriaxone induced pseudolithiasis are asymptomatic and detected on sonography. If cholelithiasis is symptomatic, discontinuation of drug is to be done but in incidentally detected asymptomatic cases of there is no need to stop drug. Usually these sludge/stones appear after one week of therapy and disappear after two weeks of discontinuation of therapy, however the time duration may vary with patient [34, 35].

2.6 Genetics

Various lithogenic gene variants have been found linked to formation of gall stones. Genome-wide association study (GWAS) have found a hepatobiliary cholesterol transporter ABCG8 [p.D19H] as the most common genetic risk factor for gall stones [36]. Mutations in the ABCB4, ABCB11, CFTR [cystic fibrosis transmembrane conductance regulator] CYP7A1 gene causes gallstones by alteration in bile composition and secretion. Gall stone has been reported as initial symptom in early

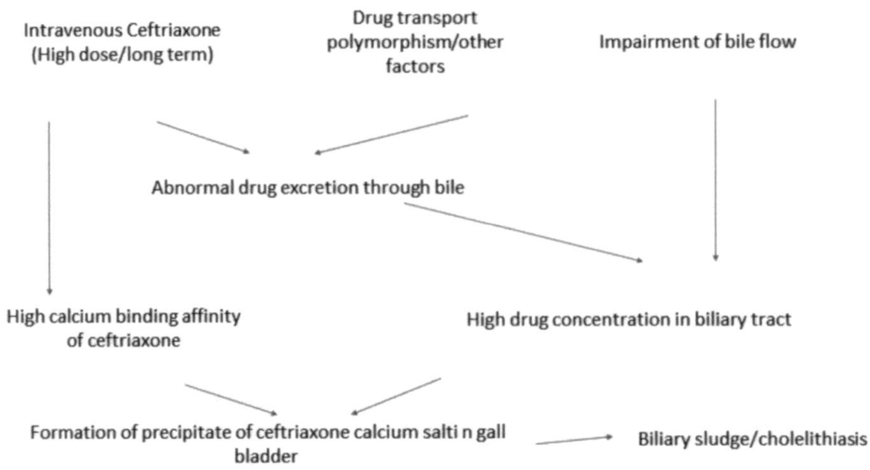

Figure 1.
Ceftriaxone induced pseudolithiasis.

childhood due to compound heterozygous mutation in ABCB4 gene (linked to progressive familial intrahepatic cholestasis type 3), these children are at risk of further developing decompensated chronic liver disease [37]. NPC1L1 [Niemann-Pick C1-Like 1] is responsible for intestinal and hepatobiliary cholesterol absorption. Functional studies showed that loss of function mutations of NPC1L1 are associated with decreased intestinal cholesterol absorption, changes in plasma low-density lipoprotein cholesterol levels decrease the reuptake of cholesterol from bile and thus promoting biliary cholesterol supersaturation. Gilbert promoter variant of the UDP glucuronosyl transferase gene [UGT1A1], appears to be an additional risk factor for gallstone risk. Studies have found that individuals predisposed to gall stone are characterized by an increased biliary output of cholesterol in the setting of relatively low intestinal cholesterol absorption, pointing to enhanced whole-body sterol clearance. An ethnic gradient in the ratios of phytosterols to cholesterol precursors (highest in Germans) is also apparent which correlates negatively with susceptibility to gallstones [38].

2.7 Obesity

In adults the association between obesity with cholelithiasis is well known. A higher incidence of cholelithiasis has also been noticed in obese children [39]. Obese children and those with a higher mean BMI (>21.5) are at higher risk of cholelithiasis and more symptomatic compared to children with a normal BMI [9]. It is recommended that children with biliary symptoms or cholelithiasis, as well as unclear ultrasonography of the bile ducts with a BMI of 23 or more should routinely undergo MRCP to rule out choledocholithiasis. There is mechanical hypothesis for more prevalence of choledocholithiasis in obese children which postulates that higher body fat content in the abdominal wall causes greater intra-abdominal pressure, resulting in external pressure on the wall of the gallbladder, this relatively higher pressure in the sub-hepatal region may results in a direct stimulus which further leads to dislodgment of the stone/sludge from the gallbladder into the extrahepatic biliary tree system, causing obstruction of the bile duct. The incidence of obesity in children rising in the some parts of world, the incidence of symptomatic cholelithiasis will also increase. Prevalence of cholelithiasis is significantly higher in patients with NAFLD (non-alcoholic fatty liver disease) [40].

2.8 Total parenteral nutrition and cholelithiasis

Total parenteral nutrition [TPN] impairs enterohepatic circulation and cholecystokinin induced gallbladder contraction resulting in biliary stasis, sludge and stones [41]. The risk of cholelithiasis increase with duration of TPN therapy, and if there is associated ileal resection or disease. Prolonged TPN therapy can lead to gallstones in 43% of children and it increases up to 64% in children with ileal resection or disease [42, 43]. Sludge formation occurs more rapidly in neonates with after a mean duration of 10 days of TPN infusion, as compared to adults where it takes more than 6 weeks.

3. Clinical features

Unlike adults, children are likely to be symptomatic, the prevalence of symptomatic children is from 50–70% [44]. The most common clinical presentation is right upper quadrant abdominal pain [usually after meals] which may be radiating to the right shoulder, nausea, vomiting and occasionally fever. Symptoms are more seen if cholelithiasis is associated with complications like cholestasis, cholecystitis, and cholangitis, in these settings additional symptoms like icterus and Murphy's sign can be seen. In infants, mostly cholelithiasis is asymptomatic and incidentally diagnosed on abdominal ultrasound.

3.1 Differential diagnosis of gall stones

The conditions mimicking the clinical features of cholelithiasis are gastroesophageal reflux disease, peptic ulcer disease, dyspepsia, acute acalculous cholecystitis, pancreatitis, hepatitis, irritable bowel syndrome, esophageal spasm, pneumonia, cardiac chest pain, and diabetic ketoacidosis and to be kept as differential diagnosis. A proper history and physical examination along with ultrasound imaging will help in making a final diagnosis.

4. Complications of gallstones

4.1 Acute calculous cholecystitis

Obstruction of the cystic duct by stones lead to inflammation of the gallbladder resulting in acute calculous cholecystitis. The obstruction causes gallbladder swelling followed by bile acid concentration, ischemia of gall bladder wall and occasionally, bacterial infection. Symptoms include pain similar to biliary colic with increased vomiting and fever. Patients usually have right upper quadrant tenderness on clinical examination and sometimes a palpable mass. Ultrasound can identify cholecystitis by presence of stone or sludge with gallbladder wall thickening and edema [double-wall sign], and pericholecystic fluid.

4.2 Common bile duct obstruction

The exact prevalence of choledocholithiasis in children is not known but they are uncommon in children. Common bile duct stones are mostly associated with gallstones except in few conditions like hemolysis where they can be primary. Presentation of choledocholithiasis include jaundice, acholic stools, and dark urine, sometimes presentation is with acute cholangitis, manifested by fever, jaundice, and right upper quadrant pain. Choledocholithiasis should also be suspected in a patient with gallstones with raised conjugated bilirubin and/or a dilated common bile duct [as per age] on ultrasound.

4.3 Pancreatitis

Cholelithiasis is one of the leading cause of acute pancreatitis in adults, however the exact incidence of gallstone pancreatitis in children is not known. Patients with gallstone pancreatitis present with epigastric abdominal pain, nausea, and vomiting or jaundice. Sometimes gall stones are detected on evaluation of pancreatitis only. Ultrasound should be the first imaging modality followed by CT scan in doubtful cases. Biochemical investigation shows elevated serum amylase and lipase levels, and elevated conjugated serum bilirubin is often present.

5. Investigation

Ultrasound is the most accurate imaging study to evaluate for gall stones, can detect as small as 1.5 mm. On ultrasound gallstones appears as hyperechoic, single or multiple and characteristically cast an acoustic shadow in contrast biliary sludge appears echogenic on ultrasound, but does not cast an acoustic shadow. Both sensitivity and specificity of ultrasonography is 95% for gall stones, but it is low for stones in common bile duct [45]. Cholescintigraphy, with Tc 99 m labeled diisopropyl iminodiacetic acid [DISIDA], is the most accurate method of diagnosing acute cholecystitis, non-visualization of the gallbladder in an otherwise patent biliary system suggests acute cholecystitis. Magnetic resonance cholangiopancreatography (MRCP) is being used increasingly to investigate complicated gallstone disease and choledocholithiasis and for delineating pancreatic and biliary tract anatomy. Endoscopic retrograde cholangiopancreatography (ERCP) can be done for both diagnostic and therapeutic in common bile duct stones. Endoscopic ultrasound can be used for diagnosis in children with complicated biliary stone disease CT scan do not have much role in diagnosis of gall stones [46, 47]. There are no specific laboratory tests in diagnosing cholelithiasis, some blood tests are required for making etiological diagnosis and to rule out complications. These include Complete blood count, liver function tests, lipid profile [serum cholesterol (LDL, HDL, VLDL) and serum triglycerides], hemolytic profile [reticulocytes, osmotic fragility, quantitative glucose 6 phosphate dehydrogenase (G6PD) measurement, hemoglobin electrophoresis, direct coombs test], next generation sequencing (if genetic cause suspected) and sweat chloride test (if cystic fibrosis suspected) and serum amylase and lipase, if pancreatitis is suspected.

6. Management

Management of cholelithiasis is affected by several contributing factors, such as type of stone, anatomical status of gallstone, rate of symptoms in the child, underlying anatomical malformations, other underlying disease, inflammatory changes of the biliary system, and age of the child. Children with gallstones should be divided into two groups, symptomatic and asymptomatic. Symptomatic and complicated gallstones need cholecystectomy [48]. Gallstones which float in the gallbladder, having a diameter of less than 10 mm and are diagnosed incidentally in asymptomatic children, should be investigated for haemolytic diseases and underlying disorders and need to be treated after diagnosis. In infants mostly, cholelithiasis resolves after several months of monitoring. However, cholelithiasis is not usually resolved spontaneously in older children. In a prospective study of children with nonpigmented gallstones it was found that, 50% remained or became asymptomatic, 32% experienced definite improvement in symptoms, and 18% had continued symptoms but none had any biliary complications [49]. The risk of subsequent hospital admission in children and adolescents with cholelithiasis increases by 5% for every 10 days [50]. Also, one fourth of children with gall stones, presents directly with complications [51]. Therapy with UDCA is recommended in asymptomatic patients with cholesterol stones [52]. However, the role of dissolution therapy in the management of gallstones in children remains to be defined, the use of UDCA therapy is restricted due to the long course of treatment, differential outcome, and the risk of side-effects such as diarrhea and liver dysfunction [53]. Gallstones when located in the common bile duct or around the pupillary sphincter, can cause cholangitis, obstruction of bile flow, and jaundice, stone removal should be done urgently tp relieve obstruction. In centres where pediatric ERCP is offered the endoscopic approach to relieve obstruction is safe and effective, if not laparoscopic exploration is also safe and effective alternative. In recent years, laparoscopic cholecystectomy (LC) has become the treatment of choice in the surgical management of children with cholelithiasis. Approach for mnagemement of gall stones in children given in **Figure 2**. LC is less invasive, has lower morbidity and mortality with shorter hospital stay in comparison to conventional open cholecystectomy [54]. Extracorporeal shock-wave lithotripsy is another therapeutic method, in selective cases like when the patient is asymptomatic or with the radiolucent gallstone.

In children receiving TPN especially longer duration should be assessed for gallstones. On discontinuation of TPN regimen and start of oral diet leads to establishment of bile flow which resolves bile sedimentation. TPN needs to be continued in cases where enteral feeding cant be done such as intestinal pseudo-obstruction or short bowel syndrome, in these patients therapeutic cholecystectomy should be done in presence of gallstones [55].

The approach to cholelithiasis in infancy is different as spontaneous resolution has been reported in a significant proportion of cases (cholelithiasis~50% and choledocholithiasis~30%). Spontaneous resolution within 6 months is more common

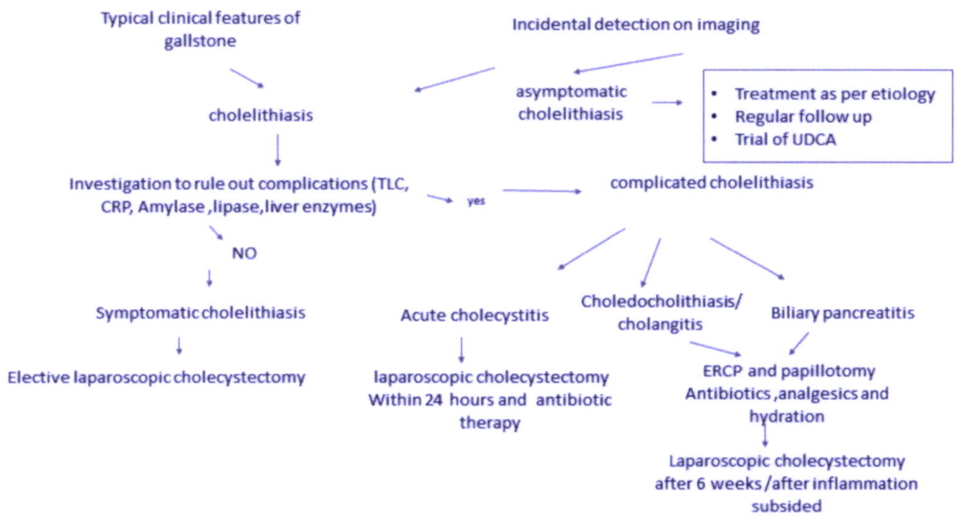

Figure 2.
Approach for management of gallstones in children.

with idiopathic and or asymptomatic gallstones than in patients with known predisposing factors. Cholecystectomy is indicated for symptomatic cholelithiasis, asymptomatic cholelithiasis persisting beyond 12 months and radiopaque calculi [56, 57].

6.1 Management of cholelithiasis in hemolytic disease

In children with hemolytic anaemias, screening for gall stones with Ultrasound is recommended from 5 years of age. Screening is also recommended before splenectomy as both splenectomy and cholecystectomy to be done in single setting in presence of gallstones [58, 59]. In sickle-cell disease, prophylactic cholecystectomy is recommended even for asymptomatic gallstones as it is difficult to differentiate an acute abdominal crisis from acute cholecystitis, and the morbidity and mortality of emergency cholecystectomy in acute crisis is much higher than in elective cholecystectomy [58]. To avoid sickling during the perioperative period hypotension, hypoxia, hypothermia, dehydration, and acidosis should be avoided and hemoglobin S should be kept below 30% and total hemoglobin should be at least of 11 g/dL [60, 61]. Many studies recommended LC in asymptomatic patients with hemolytic diseases to avoid the complications of urgent cholecystectomy and the chance of gallstone complications among the asymptomatic patients is upto 50% within 5 year of diagnosis [62]. Inflammation and infection of the gallbladder also increases the chance of a hemolytic crisis. Oral hydroxyurea reduces the frequency of cholelithiasis in some haemolytic diseases, such as thalassemia intermedia or major.

7. Prevention of gall stones

Gallstones are formed due to interaction of multiple factors like genetic, anatomical, systemic and metabolic abnormalities. However, there are some preventive factors especially for cholesterol gallstones which include regular diet, lifestyle, physical exercise, and intake of vitamin C. Lifestyle should include physical activity, ideal weight maintenance and weight reduction among overweight and obese children to prevent gall stones. It has been found that physical activity decreases the risk of symptomatic stones by about 30–70%. Regular exercise reduces insulin levels, insulin resistance, triglyceridemia, and fatty acid-dependent hypersecretion of gallbladder mucin. Also, physical activity has a prokinetic effect on the intestine and cholecystokinin-dependent gallbladder contraction. High fiber and regular eating pattern diets decrease hydrophobic bile acids, and reduces gallbladder stasis by increasing gallbladder emptying. Regular vitamin C supplementation or diet containing higher amount of vitamin C have a protective effect on gallstone formation. Situations associated with rapid loss of weight like very low-calorie diet or bariatric surgery, temporary oral UDCA may be recommended to prevent gall stone formation as the risk of cholelithiasis is much higher in these situations. There is also some role of fish oil polyunsaturated fatty acids on prevention of gall stones in obese patients. In sickle cell anemia hydroxyurea has been found to have some preventive role for pigment stones.

Conflict of interest

The author declare no conflict of interest.

DOI: http://dx.doi.org/10.5772/intechopen.99020

Author details

Nida Mirza Shaikh
Sri Aurbindo Institute of Medical Sciences, Indore, India

*Address all correspondence to: nydamirza.1@gmail.com

References

[1] Poddar U. Gallstone disease in children. Indian Pediatr. 2010 Nov;47(11):945-953. doi:10.1007/s13312-010-0159-2. PMID: 21149901.

[2] Wesdorp I, Bosman D, de Graaff A, Aronson D, van der Blij F, Taminiau J. Clinical presentations and predisposing factors of cholelithiasis and sludge in children. J Pediatr Gastroenterol Nutr. 2000;31(4):411-7.[PubMed: 11045839)

[3] Bogue CO, Murphy AJ, Gerstle JT, Moineddin R, Daneman A. Risk factors, complications, and outcomes of gallstones in children: A single-center review. J Pediatr Gastroenterol Nutr. 2010;50(3):303-308. doi: 10.1097/MPG.0b013e3181b99c72 [PubMed: 20118803].

[4] Wyllie R, Hyams JS, Kay M. Pediatric Gastrointestinal and Liver Disease. 5th ed. Philadelphia, PA: Elsevier; 2016.

[5] Vegunta RK, Raso M, Pollock J, Misra S, Wallace LJ, Torres AJ, et al. Biliary dyskinesia: The most common indication for cholecystectomy in children. Surgery. 2005;138(4):726-731. doi: 10.1016/j.surg.2005.06.052 [PubMed: 16269302].

[6] Svensson J, Makin E. Gallstone disease in children. Semin Pediatr Surg. 2012 Aug;21(3):255-265. doi: 10.1053/j.sempedsurg.2012.05.008. PMID: 22800978

[7] Portincasa P, Moschetta A, Berardino M, Di-Ciaula A, Vacca M, Baldassarre G, et al. Impaired gallbladder motility and delayed orocecal transit contribute to pigment gallstone and biliary sludge formation in beta-thalassemia major adults. World J Gastroenterol. 2004;10(16):2383-90 [PubMed: 15285024].

[8] Hussaini SH, Pereira SP, Veysey MJ, Kennedy C, Jenkins P, Murphy GM, et al. Roles of gall bladder emptying and intestinal transit in the pathogenesis of octreotide induced gall bladder stones. Gut 1996;38: 775-783.

[9] Angelico M, Gandin C, Canuzzi P, Bertasi S, Cantafora A, De Santis A, et al. Gallstones in cystic fibrosis: a critical reappraisal. Hepatology. 1991;14(5):768-75 [PubMed: 1937382].

[10] Stringer MD, Taylor DR, Soloway RD. Gallstone composition: are children different?. J Pediatr. 2003;142(4):435-440 [PubMed: 12712064].

[11] Gallbladder, Gallstones, And diseases of the Gallbladder in children Deborah a. Goldman, MD* *Pediatric institute, Cleveland Clinic Foundation, Cleveland, OH.

[12] Schweizer P, Lenz MP, Kirschner HJ. Pathogenesis and symptomatology of cholelithiasis in childhood. Dig Surg 2000; 17: 459-467

[13] Al-Mulhim AS, Abdulatif MM, Ali AM. Laparoscopic cholecystectomy in children with sickle cell disease. Saudi J Gastroenterol. 2006;12(3):130.

[14] Webb DK, Darby JS, Dunn DT, Terry SI, Serjeant GR. Gallstones in Jamaican children with homozygous sickle-cell disease. Arch Dis Child 1989; 64: 693-696.

[15] Tripathy D, Dash BP, Mohapatra BN, Kar BC. Cholelithiasis in sickle cell disease in India. J Assoc Physicians India 1997; 45: 287-289.

[16] Do Santos Gumiero AP, Bellomo-Brandao MA, Costa-Pinto EAL. Gallstones in children with sickle cell disease followed up at a Brazilian hematology center. Arq Gastroenterol 2008; 45: 313-318.

[17] Manciu S, Matei E, Trandafir B. Hereditary Spherocytosis - Diagnosis, Surgical Treatment and Outcomes. A Literature Review. Chirurgia (Bucur). 2017 Mar-Apr;112(2):110-116. doi: 10.21614/chirurgia.112.2.110. PMID: 28463670.

[18] Croom RD 3rd, McMillan CW, Orringer EP, Sheldon GF. Hereditary spherocytosis. Recent experience and current concept of pathophysiology. Ann Surg 1986; 203: 34-39.

[19] Kar R, Rao S, Srinivas UM, Mishra P, Pati HP. Clinico-hematological profile of hereditary spherocytosis: Experience from a tertiary care center in North India. Hematology 2009; 14: 164-167.

[20] Kalayci AG, Albayrak D, Gunes M, Incesu L, Agac R. The incidence of gallbladder stones and gallbladder function in beta-thalassemic children. Acta Radiol 1999; 40: 440-443.

[21] Lotfi M, Keramati P, Assadsangabi R, Nabavizadeh SA, Karimi M. Ultrasonographic assessment of the prevalence of cholelithiasis and biliary sludge in beta-thalassemia patients in Iran. Med Sci Monit 2009; 15; CR398-CR402.

[22] Origa R, Galanello R, Perseu L, Tavazzi D, Cappellini MD, Terenzani L, et al. Cholelithiasis in thalassemia major. Eur J Hematol 2008; 82: 22-25.

[23] Banerjee, S.; Owen, C.; Chopra, S. Sickle cell hepatopathy. Hepatology 2001, 33, 1021-1028.

[24] Gardner, K.; Suddie, A.; Kane, P.; O'Grady, J.; Heaton, N.; Bomford, A.; Thein, S.L. How we treat sickle hepatopathy and liver transplantation in adults. Blood 2014, 123, 2302-2307.

[25] Schaad UB, Tschappeler H, Lentze MJ. Transient formation of precipitations in the gallbladder associated with ceftriaxone therapy. Pediatr Infect Dis 1986; 5: 708-710.

[26] Rosmorduc O, Hermelin B, Poupon R. MDR3 gene defect in adults with symptomatic intrahepatic and gallbladder cholesterol cholelithiasis. Gastroenterology 2001; 120: 1449-1467.

[27] Beretsky I, Lankin DH. Diagnosis of fetal cholelithiasis using real-time high resolution imaging employing digital detection. J Ultrasound Med 1983; 2: 381-383.

[28] Suma V, Marini A, Bucci N, Toffolutti T, Talenti E. Fetal gallstones: Sonographic and clinical observations. Ultrasound Obstet Gynecol 1998; 12: 439-441.

[29] Brown LD, Teele LR, Doubilet MP. Echogenic material in the fetal gallbladder: Sonographic and clinical observations. Radiology 1992; 182: 73-76.

[30] Abbitt LP, Mc Ilhenuy J. Prenatal detection of gallstones. J Clin Ultrasound 1990; 18: 202-204.

[31] Richards DM, Heel RC, Brogden RN, Speight TM, Avery GS. Ceftriaxone. A review of its antibacterial activity, pharmacological properties and therapeutic use. Drugs 1984; 27: 469-527.

[32] Shiffman ML, Keith FB, Moore EW. Pathogenesis of ceftriaxone-associated biliary sludge. In vitrostudies of calcium-ceftriaxone binding and solubility. Gastroenterology 1990; 99: 1772-1778.

[33] Lee SP, Lipsky BA, Teefey SA. Gallbladder sludge and antibiotics. Pediatr Infect Dis J 1990; 9: 422-423.

[34] Schaad UB, Wedgwood-Krucko J, Tschaeppeler H. Reversible ceftriaxone-associated biliary pseudolithiasis in children. Lancet 1988; 2: 1411-1413.

[35] Schaad UB, Suter S, Gianella-Borradori A, Pfenninger J,

Auckenthaler R, Bernath O, et al. A comparison of ceftriaxone and cefuroxome for the treatment of bacterial meningitis in children. N Engl J Med 1990; 322: 141-147.

[36] Buch Set al. A genome-wide association scan identifies the hepatic cholesterol transporter ABCG8 as a susceptibility factor for human gallstone disease. Nat Genet. 2007;39:995-999.

[37] Mirza N, Malhotra S, Sibal A. A novel compound heterozygous mutation in ABCB4 gene leading to Cholelithiasis, progressive familial intrahepatic cholestasis (type 3), and cirrhosis in a child. J Child Sci 2020;10:e134–e136.

[38] Rebholz C, Krawczyk M, Lammert F. Genetics of gallstone disease. Eur J Clin Invest. 2018 Jul;48(7):e12935. doi: 10.1111/eci.12935. Epub 2018 May 9. PMID: 29635711.

[39] Krawczyk M, Portincasa P, Lammert F. Predictive serum markers of gallstone disease: Gazing into a Crystall ball. J. Pediatr. Gastroenterol. Nutr. 2017;64:337-338

[40] Koebnick C, Smith N, Black MH, Porter AH., Richie BA, Hudson S, et al: Pediatric obesity and gallstone disease: Results from a cross-sectional study of over 510,000 youth. J Pediatr Gastroenterol Nutr., 2012: 5(3): 328.

[41] Jaruvongvanich V, Sanguankeo A, Upala S: Significant association between gallstone disease and nonalcoholic fatty liver disease: a systematic review and meta-analysis. Digestive diseases and sciences 61.8 (2016): 2389±2396. doi:10.1007/s10620-016-4125-2 PMID: 26993825

[42] Jawaheer G, Pierro A, Lloyd DA, Shaw NJ. Gallbladder contractility in neonates: Effects of parenteral and enteral feeding. Arch Dis Child Fetal Neonatal Ed 1995; 72: F200-F202.

[43] Roslyn JJ, Berquist WE, Pitt HA, Mann LL, Kangarloo H, DenBesten L, Ament ME. Increased risk of gallstones in children receiving total parenteral nutrition. Pediatrics 1983; 71: 784-789

[44] Enayet, A., Afifi, R.A., Mogahed, E.A. et al. Gallstones in Egyptian infants and children: Risk factors, complications and outcome: A single center experience. Egypt Liver Journal 10, 31 (2020). doi:10.1186/s43066-020-00037-9

[45] Millar AJW. Surgical disorders of the liver and bile ducts and portal hypertension. In: Kelly DA editors, Disease of the Liver and Biliary System in Children, 3rd Edition, Wiley-Blackwell Publication UK, 2008, pp. 433-474.

[46] Poddar U, Thapa BR, Bhasin DK, Prasad A, Nagi B, Singh K. Endoscopic retrograde cholangiopancreatography in the management of pancreatobiliary disorders in children. J Gastroenterol Hepatol 2001; 16: 927-931.

[47] Prasad H, Poddar U, Thapa BR, Bhasin DK, Singh K. Endoscopic management of post laparoscopic cholecystectomy bile leak in a child. Gastrointest Endosc 2000; 51: 506-507.

[48] Diez S, Müller H, Weiss C, Schellerer V, Besendörfer M. Cholelithiasis and cholecystitis in children and adolescents: Does this increasing diagnosis require a common guideline for pediatricians and pediatric surgeons?. BMC Gastroenterol. 2021;21(1):186. Published 2021 Apr 21. doi:10.1186/s12876-021-01772-y

[49] Bruch SW, Ein SH, Rocchi C, Kim PCW. The management of nonpigmented gallstones in children. J Pediatr Surg 2000; 35: 729-732.

[50] Sarrami M, Ridley W, Nightingale S, Wright T, Kumar R. Adolescent gallstones-need for early intervention in

symptomatic idiopathic gallstones. Pediatr Surg Int. 2019;35(5):569-574.

[51] Tannuri AC, Leal AJ, Velhote MC, Gonlcalves ME, Tannuri U. Management of gallstone disease in children: A new protocol based on the experience of a single center. J Pediatr Surg. 2012;47(11):2033-2038.

[52] Gutt C et al. Updated S3-guideline for prophylaxis, diagnosis and treatment of gallstones. German society for digestive and metabolic diseases (DGVS) and German Society for Surgery of the Alimentary Tract (DGAV)—AWMF Registry 021/008. Z Gastroenterol. 2018;56(8):912-66

[53] Gamba PG, Zancan L, Muraca M, Vilei MT, Talenti E, Guglielmi M. is there a place of medical treatment in children with gallstones? J Pediatr Surg 1997; 32: 476-478.

[54] Chan S, Currie J, Malik AI, Mahomed AA. Pediatric cholecystectomy: Shifting goalposts in the laparoscopic era. Surg Endosc 2008; 22: 1392-1395.

[55] Matos C, Avni EF, Van Gansbeke D, Pardou A, Struyven J. Total parenteral nutrition (TPN) and gallbladder diseases in neonates. Sonographic assessment. J Ultrasound Med. 1987;6(5):243-248 [PubMed: 3108519].

[56] Debray D, Pariente D, Gauthier F, Myara A, Bernard O. Cholelithiasis in infancy: A study of 40 cases. J Pediatr 1993; 122: 385-391.

[57] Holcomb GW Jr, Holcomb GW III. Cholelithiasis in infants, children and adolescents. Pediatric Rev 1990; 11: 268-274

[58] Marchetti M, Quaglini S, Barosi G. Prophylactic splenectomy and cholecystectomy in mild hereditary spherocytosis: Analyzing the decision in different clinical scenarios. J Intern Med 1998; 244: 217-226.

[59] Sandler A, Winkel G, Kimura K, Soper R. The role of prophylactic cholecystectomy during splenectomy in children with hereditary spherocytosis. J Pediatr Surg 1999; 34: 1077-1078.

[60] Al-Salem AH. Should cholecystectomy be performed concomitantly with splenectomy in children with sickle-cell disease? Pediatr Surg Int 2003; 19: 71-74.

[61] Muroni M, Loi V, Lionnet F, et al. Prophylactic laparoscopic cholecystectomy in adult sickle cell disease patients withcholelithiasis: A prospective cohort study. Int J Surg. 2015;22:62-66.

[62] Curro G, Meo A, Ippolito D, et al. Asymptomatic cholelithiasis in children with sickle cell disease: Early or delayed cholecystectomy? Ann Surg. 2007;245(1):126-129.

Chapter 2

Minimally Invasive Treatment for Cholelithiasis

Hirotaka Okamoto

Abstract

Gallstone disease, cholecysto- and choledocho-lithiasis, is one of the most common digestive diseases. Most patients with symptomatic cholecystolithiasis are recommended to undergo cholecystectomy to alleviate their symptoms like abdominal pain and jaundice. Approximately 10–20% of patients who undergo cholecystectomy for gallstones have choledocholithiasis. Nowadays, endoscopic and/or laparoscopic approaches are widely accepted as the treatment for patients with gallstone. Patients with cholecystolithiasis are usually treated by laparoscopic cholecystectomy, whereas patients with choledocholithiasis are done by endoscopic sphincterotomy (EST) or laparoscopic common bile duct exploration (LCBDE). Additionally, some cases are treated by biliary reconstruction such as biliary enteric anastomosis. In this chapter, currently available laparoscopic approaches as a minimally invasive surgery are introduced and discussed on the basis of pathogenesis of the gallstone.

Keywords: minimal invasive surgery, laparoscopic cholecystectomy, lapatoscopic biliary enteric anastomosis

1. Introduction

Gallstone disease is one of the most common and popular diseases. The prevalence of this disease estimates to be approximately 10% of the adult population. Most patients are asymptomatic, but a certain percentage of patients are symptomatic. Operation of biliary tree including laparoscopic cholecystectomy are among the most common abdominal operative procedures.

2. Pathogenesis of gallstones

Gallstones are classified into cholesterol stone and pigment stone. Pathogenesis of cholesterol gallstone formation is considered to consist of three elements. First is biliary stasis, second is nucleation, and third is lithogenic bile (**Figure 1**) [1]. A cause of lithogenic bile has derived from cholesterol supersaturation. Aggregation of cholesterol-phospholipid vesicles is important to nucleation and formation of cholesterol-crystal. Biliary stasis in the gallbladder has been another factor associated with an increased incidence of cholelithiasis [2]. Pigmented stones are classified as either brown or black stones. Pathogenesis of pigmented stone is considered a result of infection [3].

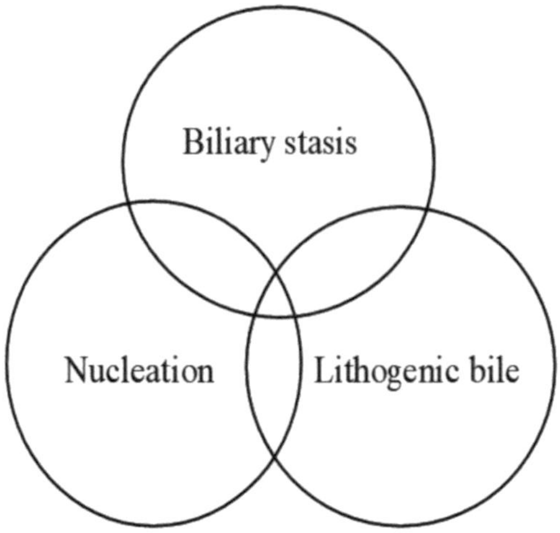

Figure 1.
Three factors of cholesterol gallstone formation.

3. Clinical manifestation

It is generally assumed that approximately more than half of all patients with gallstones are asymptomatic in the natural history. The remaining patients may have intermitted histories of biliary colic pain, or presenting with acute cholecystitis, symptom following to choledocholithiasis or gall stone pancreatitis. Of them, only small percentages of patients with symptomatic gallstone disease developed serious complication within a certain period [4]. One of potential risks of patients with gallstone disease is the development of gallbladder carcinoma [5, 6].

3.1 Acute cholecystitis

Acute inflammation of the gallbladder is the most frequent complication of gallstone disease. The initiating factor is the stone impaction either cystic duct or in the infundibulum of the gallbladder. It is frequently explored for intra-abdominal emergency, in particularly in middle-aged women and in the elderly. Approximately more than 50% of patients with acute cholecystitis have been bacteria in the bile culture, but these factors are thought to play a secondary role in the pathogenesis of cholecystitis. Bacteria typically isolated are of enteric origin, with the most common species being, *Escherichia coli*. Other bacteria may be present include Enterobacter, Klebsiella, or Enterococcus. Morphological changes of acute cholecystitis include, edema, hypervascularity, venous congestion, gallbladder distension.

3.2 Chronic cholecystitis

Whereas bacteria can be cultured from the bile of approximately more than 50% of patients with acute cholecystitis, the incidence of positive bile cultures in patients with chronic cholecystitis is less than 20%. In patients who have had recurring biliary colic pain with long-term gallstones, some of them had fibrosis and small round cell infiltration with the gallbladder wall thickening. Some patients with recurring biliary colic pain are thought histologically to have chronic cholecystitis.

4. Operative management of cholecystolithiasis

Historically, surgical technique of cholecystolithotomy, removing the gallstone from bladder and leaving the organ in the body, was firstly introduced by John Bobbs, an Indiana surgeon in the late 1800s. However, this procedure was not effective, because recurrence of symptom with the stone had occurred. Thereafter, open cholecystectomy (OC) had been introduced for gallstone disease by Karl Langenbuch, a German surgeon in 1882 [7]. Since then, this open surgery has become the gold standard for the management of patients with symptomatic gallstone over a 100 year. The introduction of laparoscopic cholecystectomy (LC) has revolutionized approach to patients with symptomatic gallstone disease in 1988 [8, 9]. This minimal invasive approach has soon emerged and spread world-widely for the patients with uncomplicated cholelithiasis and cholecystitis [10–12].

5. Laparoscopic cholecystectomy (LC)

5.1 Indications and contraindications of LC

The presence of symptomatic gallstones with biliary colic pain, intermittent right upper quadrant or epigastric pain, radiated pain with or without nausea and vomiting is the primary indication for LC. Complication of gallstones are acute cholecystitis, obstructive jaundice, and pancreatitis, is also indication of cholecystectomy. Patients with acute cholecystitis should be performed urgent LC within 72 hours. Patients with acute phase longer than 72 hours are likely to have a significant dense and inflammatory adhesion, so that some surgeons prefer to perform an initial conservative management of the disease, followed by scheduled interval cholecystectomy several week later.

Contraindication of LC includes suspicious case of gallbladder cancer, uncontrolled bleeding case, and no identified case of anatomical structure. Conversion to open laparotomy should consider in the cases of inability of definitive identification of surgical anatomy, or bleeding or bowel injury.

5.2 Anatomy

5.2.1 Hepato-cystic triangle and Calot's triangle

The hepato-cystic triangle is the space bordered by the inferior edge of the liver, the common hepatic duct, and the cystic duct of a gallbladder. The cystic artery passes through this space. The Calot's triangle is the bordered by the cystic duct, the cystic artery, and the common hepatic duct. It is important to obtain "the critical view of safety", which first described by Strasberg, et al. to avoid the common bile duct and hepatic duct injury during LC (**Figure 2**) [13].

5.3 Surgical procedure

5.3.1 Patient positioning

The patient is placed in the supine position on the operation table. The operation surgeon stands to the patient's left, scope holder to surgeon's left (British or American style) or between patient's legs (French or European style), and the assistant on the patient's right.

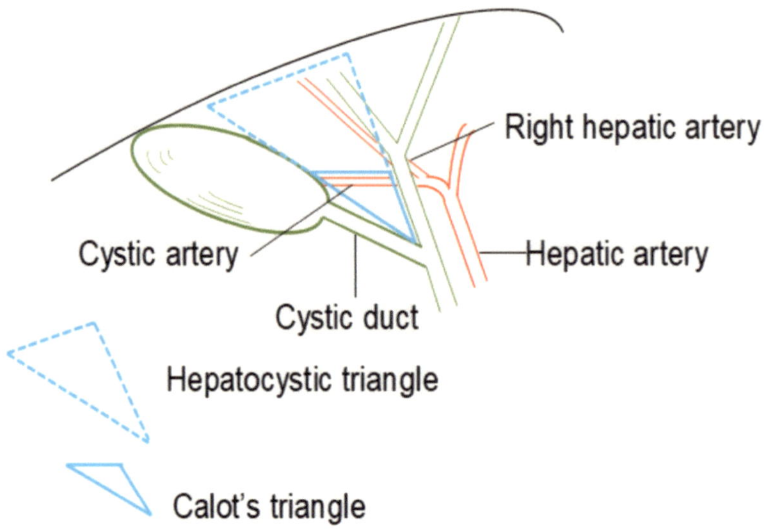

Figure 2.
Hepato-cystic triangle and Calot's triangle.

5.3.2 Port placement and pneumoperitoneum

The first 12 mm trocar is inserted through 10-15 mm incision through the umbilicus for the development of pneumoperitoneum as well as for the safe insertion of additional trocars under direct laparoscopic vision. Carbon dioxide has been used for the pneumoperitoneum in laparoscopic surgery. Abdominal pressure needs to be adjusted up to obtain adequate working-space, or down to limit the deleterious physiologic effects of the pneumoperitoneum. Abdominal pressure usually adjusts with range from 8 to 12 mmHg, avoiding a pressure about 15 mmHg. After pneumoperitoneum, laparoscope is placed through the umbilical trocar to confirm operative working space and insertion of the accessary trocars under laparoscopic view.

A total of four trocars are essential to perform a cholecystectomy. A trocar of 5 mm for grasping the fundus of the gallbladder is placed in the right anterior axillary line. A second port of 12 mm is placed high in the epigastrium, adjacent to the right of the falciform ligament. The fourth port of 5 mm is placed just below the liver edge in the right midclavicular line.

5.3.3 The dissection of the Calot's triangle

Dissection of the triangle of Calot's is the dangerous part of the operation. Critical view of safety is the important to avoid misorientation of the anatomy. A surgeon can be certain that cystic duct and cystic artery are identified only by achieving this critical view. Once identification of cystic duct, the duct is dissected only to allow the safe placement of two clips and division. Cystic artery is located cranial to the duct and usually runs paralleled to it. The cystic artery is related posterior to the sentinel lymph node, serving a useful landmark. The right hepatic artery can run very close to the gallbladder and can be easily misoriented for the cystic artery. After division of the cystic duct and artery, the gallbladder is then dissected from the liver bed. Appropriate direct- and counter-traction of gallbladder can help the gallbladder dissect from liver bed. The dissected gallbladder is extracted under direct vision through the umbilical trocar inserted site.

5.4 Complications of LC

Trocar injury to the bowel, mesentery, or vessels is care point of LC, but an insertion of the first trocar through 10-15 mm incision through the umbilicus can avoid these injuries.

A safe insertion of additional trocars under direct laparoscopic vision can also avoid these injuries. Bleeding from liver bed is among the complications. In most cases, bleeding from liver bed can be controlled with electrocautery. Bile leaks can be observed about 1% of LC cases after discharge hospital within 7 days. The cystic duct is the most common site and the bile duct is possible to occur. Once a bile leak is confirmed, percutaneous drainage and endoscopic sphincterotomy with stenting.

5.5 Advantages and disadvantages of LC

The advantages of LC are shown in **Table 1**. Postoperative pain is reduced by small size incisions of LC. The small size of the fascial incisions also allows quick return to surgical physical stress. The small incisions are also cosmetical benefits than the larger incisions of traditional open cholecystectomy. Magnified views achieved by a laparoscopy allow surgeons to inspect a precise anatomy. The patient can be recovered and discharged from the hospital and return to full activity within a few days.

However, there are several potential disadvantages of LC compared to OC (**Table 2**).

Laparoscopy has limitation of two-dimensional monocular image in contrast to three-dimensional depth perception. The operative field view is directed by a surgeon other than operator. It is more difficult to control significant hemorrhage using laparoscopy than in an open surgical view. Laparoscopic instrument has less tactile discrimination in contrast to direct digital palpation of OC. The

Less pain
Smaller incisions
Better cosmetics
Magnified view of anatomy
Earlier recover from surgical stress
Shorter hospital stay

Table 1.
Advantages of LC compared to OC.

Lack of three-dimensional perception
Views controlled by a scope holder
Control hemorrhage
Less tactile discrimination
CO_2 insufflation complication
Limit use of sever adhesion/inflammation case
Potential duct injury
Cost

Table 2.
Disadvantages of LC compared to OC.

pneumoperitoneum created by CO2 insufflation is sometimes associated with a patient systemic circulation. Generally, operation times is longer than for a conventional OC.

6. Choledocholithiasis

6.1 Pathogenesis and classification

Common bile duct stones have been noted in 10–19% of patients with cholelithiasis, and this incidence increases to about 80% with age over 90 years old [14]. Choledocholithiasis usually results from dropped stone of the gallbladder and passed through the cystic duct. These secondary bile duct stones are cholesterol stones in most cases and black stones in certain cases. These characteristic stones are formed in the presence of cholesterol saturation, nucleating factors, and biliary stasis. On the contrary, primary bile duct stones are associated with biliary stasis and infection of bacteria [15].

6.2 Clinical manifestation

Patients with choledocholithiasis may present with biliary colic, bile duct obstruction, bilirubinuria, pruritis, jaundice. Nausea and vomiting with intermittent or constant epigastric or right upper quadrant pain are occurred in cases of early phase of the biliary obstruction [16]. The clinical course may be complicated by acute gallstone pancreatitis, cholangitis, or rarely, hepatic abscess.

6.2.1 Cholangitis

Cholangitis is the most rapid fatal complication of gallstones and occurs resulting from biliary tree bacteria infection in the setting of biliary tree obstruction.

Bile duct obstruction including bile duct stone impaction results in decreased antibacterial defenses, allowing bacteria to gain access to the biliary tree. As biliary pressure rises with obstruction, bacteria with endotoxins leak into the systemic circulation and cause the sepsis [17]. Mortality of this condition approaches approximately 100% if the patients subject to needed drainage interventions [18]. Early diagnosis and immediate treatment are imperative for successful outcome.

6.2.2 Charcot's triad and Reynord's pentad

Fever, right upper quadrant pain, and jaundice is *Charcot's triad*, presenting in 50–70% of patients with cholangitis at presentation. Hypotension and altered mental status are known as *Reynold's pentad* in addition to Charcot's triad.

6.3 Treatment of cholangitis

Patients with cholangitis can become a severe condition in a short period of time, and rapid initiation of treatment is needed. Drainage of the biliary tree is the central of therapy for patients with acute cholangitis [17]. When biliary decompression by the drainage is not achieved, hepatic abscesses are unavoidable. Mortality approaches 100% in patients who are not subjected to needed drainage interventions after failure of conservative treatment [19]. Endoscopic retrograde cholangio-pancreatograph (ERCP) with bile duct clearance is a best choice of treatment of acute cholangitis and superior to the other drainage method including percutaneous transhepatic, and surgical drainage methods [20]. There are some endoscopic treatment options; The placement of naso-biliary catheters or biliary stents to sphincterotomy and stone extraction. Sphincterotomy with bile duct clearance is preferred in patients with responded to antibody therapy.

7. Operative management of cholodocholithiasis

7.1 Minimally invasive surgery

7.1.1 Laparoscopic common bile duct exploration

7.1.1.1 Transcystic duct procedure

Trans-cystic duct procedure offers a good minimally invasive approach to CBD stones. This technique can effectively avoid a choledochotomy, resulting in the complexity of intracorporeal suture closure of the CBD. In the case of multiple stones, stone proximal to the cystic duct to bile duct junction, and fragile cystic duct, this technique is not preferable. Most trans-cystic duct procedure for CBD exploration require balloon dilatation of the cystic duct. Flexible biliary endoscopy with wired basket retrieval of calculi to be the safe technique due to direct vision of wired basket manipulation and stone capture [21].

The patient positioned and ports are set in the supine position similar to laparoscopic cholecystectomy. Guidewire is placed and positioned in cystic duct in preparation for advancing a balloon dilatation catheter for cystic duct dilatation. The balloon and cystic duct are observed laparoscopically for inflation of the balloon to the insufflation pressure recommended by the manufacturer. The cystic duct should never be dilated larger than the inner diameter of the CBD. Endoscopy can be inserted over a hydrophobic guidewire gently guided with an atraumatic grasper. After the endoscopy reaches in the cystic duct and the stone is seen and surrounded by the basket, it is gently closed and the stone and scope are withdrawn together [22]. The procedure is repeated until the duct is clear. After the completion of these processes, the cystic duct stump should be closed with a clip or a loop ligature.

7.1.1.2 Choledochotomy procedure

Choledochotomy technique is preferable in the case of a dilated CBD greater than 10 mm, calculi 10 mm or larger, multiple calculi, impacted stone, or stones proximal to the cystic duct to bile duct junction. It is contraindication in a not dilated CBD because of increase difficulty and the risk of stricture. The advantages of choledochotomy are the calculi can easily be irrigated out of the CBD and an endoscopy can be inserted bidirectionally distal and proximal to bile duct. The disadvantages of choledochotomy are considerable laparoscopic suturing technique needed to close the choledochotomy wound.

The anterior wall of the CBD is dissected sharply and bluntly caring for the multiple small vessels in the area. The choledochotomy should be created in the CBD below the cystic duct and the CBD junction. Two stay sutures are placed in the CBD area, which tent the anterior wall and prevent injury to the posterior wall on incising the CBD longitudinally. The length of choledochotomy should be the same as the circumference of the largest calculi to minimize the suturing needed for closure. Introduction of the choledochoscope is done through a subcostal trocar and inserted through the choledochotomy into the CBD. A biliary wire basket or balloon catheter is used to capture and remove calculi. After finishing complete clearance of the CBD, it is possible to close the choledochotomy wound. However, concerning about large number of stones, recurrent stones, or remnant stones, surgical drainage of the CBD is needed. Surgical drainage includes T-tube drainage, choledocho-duodenostomy, or choledocho-jejunostomy.

7.1.2 Laparoscopic choledocho-duodenostomy

The common indications for choledocho-duodenostomy (CDD) are the benign diseases like impact stones with ERCP failure, retained stones, distal common bile duct stricture from chronic pancreatitis, recurrent choledocholithiasis [23, 24]. A laparoscopic CDD is typically performed by laparoscopic intracorporeal suturing, whereas a choledochojejunostomy (CJ) is done by stapled anastomosis. A CDD involves one anastomosis as compared with a CJ required as a Roux-Y limb or a jejunal loop. Another advantage of a CDD includes easy access to the biliary tree endoscopically and physiological bile drainage.

7.1.2.1 Choledochoduodenostomy procedure

The port setting for CDD is similar to the series used for a laparoscopic cholecystectomy. A flexible laparoscope or a 30-degree laparoscope is used through umbilical port. The anterior surface of the bile duct is sharply and bluntly dissected following longitudinal choledochotomy in the supra-pancreatic part of the CBD using microscissors. Incision should be made between 1.5 cm and 2.0 cm in length. After the removal of the stones, a generous Kocher's maneuver should be performed to mobilize the duodenum if needed. A longitudinal duodenostomy is made to prepare the anastomosis to the choledochotomy without tension. The posterior row of

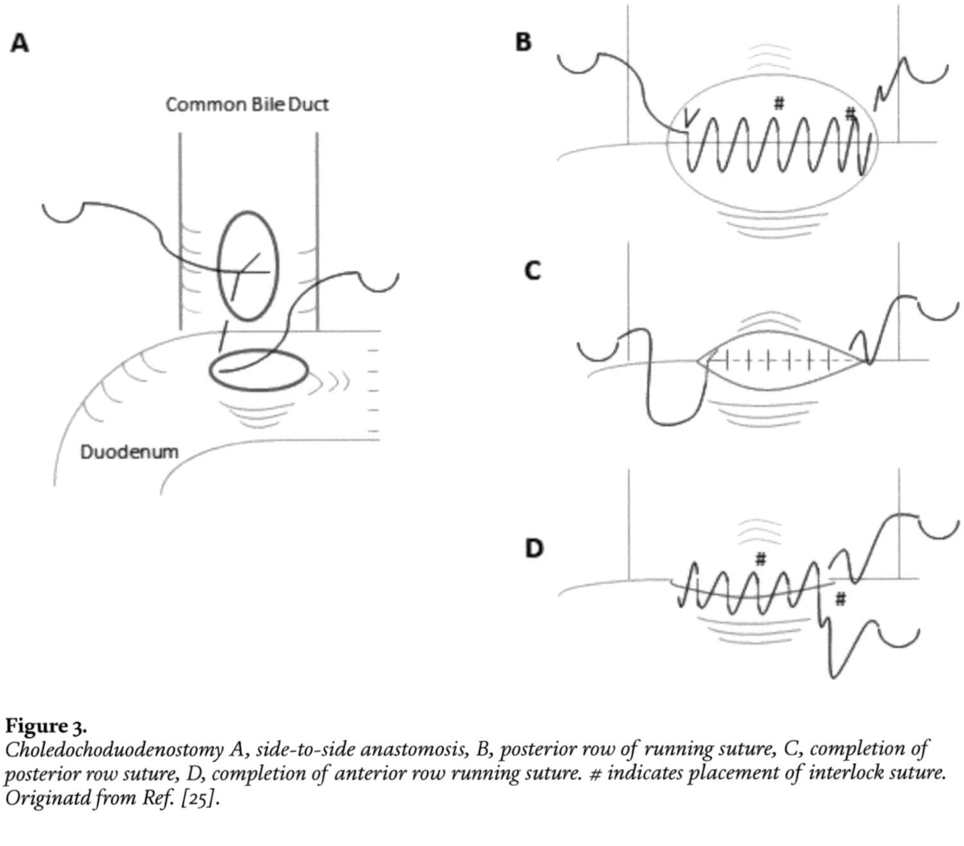

Figure 3.
Choledochoduodenostomy A, side-to-side anastomosis, B, posterior row of running suture, C, completion of posterior row suture, D, completion of anterior row running suture. # indicates placement of interlock suture. Originatd from Ref. [25].

sutures should be placed in a running fashion followed the anterior row sutures can be completed as the same fashion [25]. There are some discussions about whether a side-to-side or end-to-side anastomosis of the CDD is prefer in the laparoscopic surgery. The side-to-side anastomosis is used much often due to only requiring an anterior bile duct wall dissection. So-called "Sump syndrome" can occur with this anastomosis resulting from collecting debris or stones in distal bile duct. The end-to-side anastomosis has risks of ischemia and the stenosis due to poor blood supply of the distal bile duct (**Figure 3**).

7.1.3 Laparoscopic choledocho- or hepatioco-jejunostomy (CJ or HJ)

Laparoscopic choledocho- or hepatico-jejunostomy is a choice of biliary reconstructions when resection or exposure of the proximal bile duct or hepatic duct is required. Roux Y jejunal limb has to be created, resulting in making difficulty of the laparoscopic procedure. CJ or HJ is much advanced techniques, because of requirement of the two anastomosis of CJ or HJ with Roux-en-Y jejuno-jejunostomy.

7.1.3.1 CJ or HJ procedure

The patient is placed in supine position. The ports setting is according to laparoscopic cholecystectomy with some modification. A 5-10 mm port is added in the left mid-upper abdomen for suturing if necessary. In a case of the resection of the extra-hepatic bile duct such as a choledochal cyst, CJ or HJ should be performed because of anastomosis tension free. After the careful dissection of the bile duct along the portal vein, the duct is encircled with taping for counter-traction. The duct is dissected up to a planned point toward the duodenum and the hepatic plate followed the division using a stapling device or endoloop. Once the bile duct has been prepared, the Roux jejunal limb is created by dividing the jejunum about 20-30 cm distal to Treitz ligament with stapler. Roux Y limb passes through antecolic route and creates a side-to-side or end-to-side jejuno-jejunostomy with a stapler. CJ or HJ is performed between the bile duct and jejunal small enterostomy using a running suture on both the posterior and anterior walls of the reconstructed jejunum in the end-to-side fashion.

Author details

Hirotaka Okamoto
Department of Surgery, Tsuru Municipal Hospital, Department of Gastrointestinal, Breast and Endocrine Surgery, University of Yamanashi, Japan

*Address all correspondence to: hirotakaoka@hotmail.com

References

[1] Abedin MZ, Roslyn JJ. Gallstone pathogenesis. In Darzi A, et al, Techniques in the Management of Gallstones. Oxford, England: Blackwell Scientific; 1995.

[2] Holzbach RT. Gallbladder stasis: consequence of long-term parental hyperalimentation and risk factor for cholelithiasis. Gastroenterology 1983;84:1055.

[3] Stewart L, Smith AL, et al. Pigmented gallstones form as a composite of bacterial microcloonies and pigment solids. Ann Surg 1987;206:242.

[4] Gracie WA, Ransofhoff DF. The natural history of gallstones; the innocent gallstone is not a myth. N Engl J Med 1982;307:798.

[5] Diehl AK. Gallstone size and the risk of gallbladder cancer. JAMA 1983;250:2323-2326.

[6] Okamoto M, Okamoto H, Kitahara F, et al. Ultrasonographic evidence of association of polyps and stones with gallbladder cancer. Am J Gastroenterol 1999;94:446-450.

[7] Beal JM. Historical perspective of gallstone disease. Surg Gynecol Obstet 1984;158:181.

[8] Dubois F, Icard P, Berthelot G, et al. Coeliscopic cholecystectomy: preliminary report of 36 cases. Am J Surg 1990;211:609.

[9] Southern Surgeons club. A prospective analysis of 1,518 laparoscopic cholecystectomies. N Engl J Med 1991;324:1073.

[10] Schirmer BD, Edge SB, Dix J, et al. Laparoscopic cholercystectomy: treatment of choice for symptomatic cholelithiasis. Ann Surg 1991;213:665.

[11] Gadacz TR. U.S. experience with laparoscopic cholecystectomy. Am J Surg 1993;165:450.

[12] Kimura T, Kimura K, Katsuhiko S, et al. Laparoscopic cholecystectomy: the Japanese experience. Surg Laparosc Endosc 1993;3:194.

[13] Strasberg SM, Hertl M, Soper NJ. An analysis of the problem of biliary injury during laparoscopic cholecystectomy. J Am Coll Surg 1995;180:101-125.

[14] Tierney S, Pitt HA. Choledo cholithiasis and cholangitis. In: Bell RH, Rikkers LF, Mulholland MW (eds), Digestive Tract Surgery: A Text and Atlas. Philadelphia: Lipincott-Raven; 1996:407-431.

[15] Kaufman HS, Magnuson TH, Lillemoe KD, et al. The role of bacteria in the gallbladder and common bile duct stone formation. Ann Surg 1989;209: 584-592

[16] Faust TW, Reddy KR. Postoperative jaundice. Clin Liver Dis 2004;8:151-166.

[17] van Lent AU, Bartelsman JF, Tytgat GN, et al. Duration of antibiotics therapy for cholangitis after successful endoscopic drainage of the biliary tract. Gastrointest Endsc 2002;55:518-522.

[18] Yusoff IF, Barkun JS, Barkun AN. Diagnosis and management of cholecystitis and cholangitis. Gastroenterol Clin North Am 2003;32:1145-1168.

[19] Yusoff IF, Barkun JS, Barkun AN. Diagnosis and management of cholecystitis and cholangitis. Gastroenterol Clin North Am 2003;32 1145-1168.

[20] Bornman PC, van Beljon JI, Krige JE. Management of cholangitis. J Hepatobil Pancreat Surg 2003;10: 406-411.

[21] Hanif E, Ahmed Z, Samie E, Nassar AHM. Laparoscopic transcystic bile duct exploration: the treatment of first choice for common bile duct stones. Surg Endsc 2010;24:1552-1556.

[22] Liberman MA, Phillips EH, Carrol BJ, et al. Cost effective management of complicated choledocholithiasis: laparoscopic transcystic duct exploration or endoscopic sphincterotomy. J Am Coll Surg 1996;182:488-494.

[23] Rhodes M, Nathanson L. Laparoscopic choledochoduodenostomy. Surg Laparosc Endosc 1996;6:318-321.

[24] Tinoco R, EL-Kadre L, Tinoco A. Laparoscopic choledochoduodenostomy. J Laparoendosc Adv Surg Tech A. 1999;9:123-126.

[25] Okamoto H, Maruyama S, Takahashi K, et al. Laparoscopic choledochoduodenostomy for biliary alleviation. Surgical Science2017; 8:65-72.

Chapter 3

Routine and Innovation in Surgical Therapy of Gallstones

Peter Dubovan, Ramadan Aziri and Miroslav Tomáš

Abstract

This chapter discusses the anatomy of the gallbladder with the anatomical variations potentially impacting surgical therapy. It is dissertated upon the clinical indication for the surgical therapy with consecutive treatment. The discussion on the surgery focuses on the patient's safety and strategies for safe cholecystectomy with an optimal approach. Even though the efforts to minimise potential complications are made, the complication may arise, and therefore, the last part of this chapter discusses such cases with optimal clinical management.

Keywords: gallbladder anatomy, indication, surgical treatment, cholecystectomy, critical view of safety, complications, biliary injury

1. Introduction

The advancements in current knowledge of the human anatomy and diseases continuously led to innovation and improvements in surgical fields, with gallbladder surgery not being any different. Most of the advances were made in the last two centuries, lending the surgical pioneers perpetual reminiscence among colleagues. The names like Jean-Francois Calot, William S. Halsted, Carl Langenbuch, and others paved the way for successful gallbladder drainage and removal [1]. The introduction of open cholecystectomy led to the formation of new standards of care for the therapy of gallstones [1]. Moreover, the first video-laparoscopic gallbladder removal performed by French surgeon Philip Mouret meant the rapid spread of this new technique with majority replacement of the open surgery and changes to the state-of-the-art gallstone therapy making it in the process one of the most frequent surgeries currently performed worldwide [1, 2].

2. Anatomy of the gallbladder and the adjacent area

To perform a successful gallbladder surgery, the surgeon has to know the anatomy of this region and also be aware of potential anatomical variations resulting in a potentially more difficult surgery.

2.1 Biliary tract

Most of the time, the intrahepatic biliary ducts consecutively join forming anterior and posterior segment ducts, which drain into the right hepatic duct, and medial and lateral segment ducts draining into the left hepatic duct. The union of the right and left hepatic ducts in the porta hepatis leads to the formation of the common hepatic duct (CHD) with its distal end formed by cystic duct junction and variation in the length from 1.0 to 7.5 cm depending on the junction site with the diameter of 0.4 cm [3].

In most people, the cystic duct joins the common hepatic duct at an angle of 40° from the right side and runs parallel to the CHD for a shorter or longer distance on average for 17 mm [3]. In some cases, the cystic duct may cross the CHD posteriorly or anteriorly and join the CHD from the left side [3].

Common bile duct (CBD)/ductus choledochus is formed by the union of the CHD and the cystic duct with its distal end at the papilla of Vater in the duodenum [3]. If the cystic duct enters the duodenum separately, the common bile duct is absent [3]. Standardly the length of CBD is diverse between 5 cm and 15 cm with an average diameter of 6 mm.

Gallbladder is a pouch 7–10 cm long able to contain 30–50 ml of bile and located on the visceral liver surface in the proximity of the liver segments IV and V [3]. Liver and gallbladder are separated by the Glisson capsule's connective tissue and anteriorly, the gallbladder is covered with the peritoneum completely enfolding the *fundus* [3]. Body of the gallbladder contacts the superior and descending part of the duodenum and the transverse colon [3]. Infundibulum is the posterior part of the gallbladder body between the neck and cystic artery entrance [3]. Dilated infundibulum with a lateral bulge is called the Hartman's pouch, formerly thought to be a variation, however later regarded as a constant feature [3]. Gallbladder neck is an S-shaped narrowing continually proceeding into the cystic duct (**Figure 1**) [3].

2.2 Vasculature of the gallbladder

The blood supply to the gallbladder is secured by the cystic artery, which commonly arises from the right hepatic artery (RHA) and runs towards the gallbladder

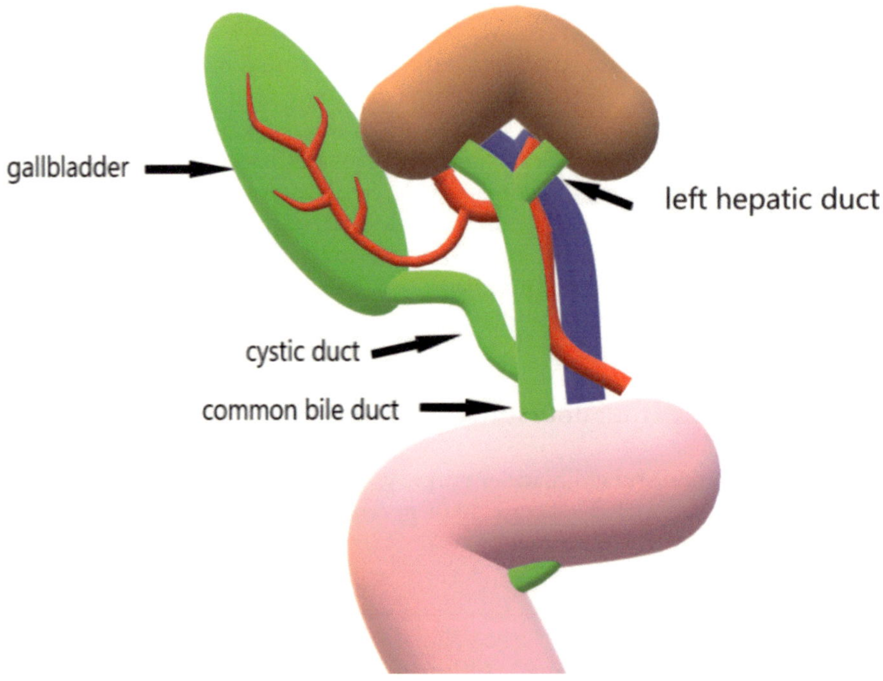

Figure 1.
Schematic image of the extrahepatic biliary tree with hepatic artery and portal vein.

just right to the common hepatic duct through the hepatocystic triangle [3]. Venous drainage is secured by a number of small veins passing through the gallbladder bed to the liver from the hepatic site, and from the peritoneal site, small veins drain into the liver through the ascending veins of the common bile duct [3]. The lymphatic drainage is secured by the collecting trunks draining into the cystic node localised in the angle between the cystic and common hepatic ducts and into the hiatal node localised on the anterior border of the epiploic foramen [3].

2.3 Hepatocystic triangle/triangle of Calot

The hepatocystic triangle is formed on the right side by the proximal part of the gallbladder and the cystic duct, on the left side by the common hepatic duct with the superior part being formed by the liver margin (**Figure 2**) [3]. Originally, the superior border of the Calot's triangle was the cystic artery; however, this area enlarged throughout the years [3]. Several structures run in the hepatocystic triangle, which have to be identified prior to any definitive surgical intervention. We have to visualise the right hepatic artery, cystic artery, common hepatic duct, and potential variations either in vascular or in biliary system [3].

2.3.1 Biliary variations in hepatocystic triangle important for gallbladder surgery

The right and left hepatic duct mostly joins at the level of the porta hepatis; however, in some individuals, this connection may be more distal eventually resulting in the absence of the common hepatic duct and potentially endangering the right hepatic duct during the surgical intervention (**Figure 3A**) [3]. Accessory hepatic duct can drain into the cystic duct or it may be mistaken for the cystic duct, and therefore, the surgeon has to be careful where to ligate the cystic duct during the surgery to preserve its function (**Figure 3C** and **D**) [3]. A similar problem arises with the duplication of the cystic duct, which may drain into the right hepatic duct, and therefore in the case of the omission of such anomaly leads to a biliary leak (**Figure 3E**) [3].

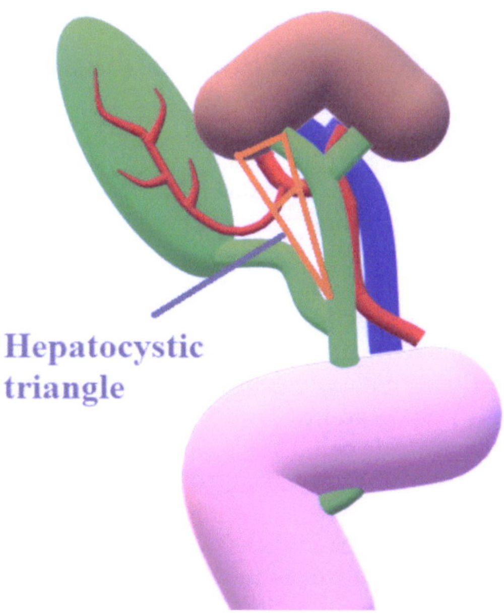

Figure 2.
Schematic image of the extrahepatic biliary tree with identified hepatocystic triangle.

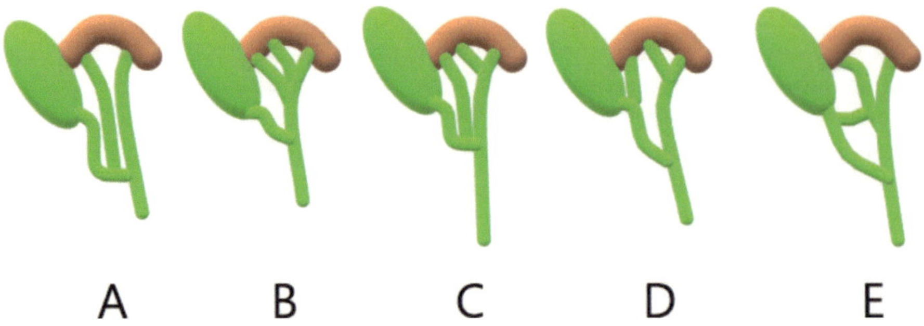

Figure 3.
Schematic image of biliary tract variations: A: distal union of the right and left hepatic duct resulting in the absence of CHD; B: accessory hepatic duct joining left hepatic duct; C: accessory hepatic duct joining distal cystic duct; D: accessory hepatic duct joining proximal cystic duct; E: accessory cystic duct joining right hepatic duct.

2.3.2 Arterial variations in hepatocystic triangle important for gallbladder surgery

The right hepatic artery (RHA) after originating from the proper hepatic artery crosses the common hepatic duct posteriorly in 85% of cases and in 15% either RHA or its branches passes anteriorly [3]. For a short distance, RHA runs parallel to the cystic artery before turning upward towards the liver and therefore can be mistaken for the cystic artery [3]. The general rule for minimising such a mistake is that no artery in the Calot's triangle with a diameter of more than 0.3 cm will be a cystic artery [3]. The superior mesenteric artery may give rise to an aberrant right hepatic artery entering the hepatocystic triangle from below and potentially giving rise to the cystic artery in the triangle [3]. In addition to the origins of the cystic artery from the right hepatic artery, there are reports describing the origins from the left hepatic artery with the course anterior to the common hepatic duct, while origins from the common hepatic artery or gastroduodenal artery mean the entry of the cystic artery to the hepatocystic triangle from below [3].

3. Indication for surgical therapy of gallstone disease

3.1 Uncomplicated gallstone disease

Individuals with the gallstone disease have in the majority of cases asymptomatic course mostly continuing throughout their lives and often are diagnosed only incidentally [4].

Therefore, asymptomatic patients do not require surgical intervention and we wait for the symptom appearance [4]. However, cholecystectomy is recommended for asymptomatic patients with an increased risk of gallbladder cancer, like those with gallstones larger than 3 cm, porcelain gallbladder, or with the presence of gallbladder adenomas [4, 5]. In addition, the surgical therapy is recommended in patients suffering from sickle cell disease and spherocytosis, if abdominal surgery is performed due to other concerns, to prevent the formation of pigment gallstones [4].

For patients, who are surgical candidates with uncomplicated gallstone disease with imaging confirmation of gallstones and symptomatic course mostly with the biliary colic, there is a recommendation for an elective surgical therapy [4]. Patients who present themselves to the emergency ward with the acute aggravation of the biliary colic are treated conservatively with planned surgical intervention after resolution of symptoms due to a lesser risk of complication in elective surgery compared to emergency surgery [4].

3.2 Complicated gallstone disease

Patients with gallstone disease affected by complications such as acute cholecystitis, cholangitis, biliary pancreatitis are recommended to undergo definitive surgical therapy.

In the treatment of acute calculous cholecystitis, it is important to correctly recognise indications for emergency surgery, which are complicated acute cholecystitis with gallbladder gangrene/necrosis, gallbladder perforation, and disease progression despite the medical therapy [6].

If the reasons for emergency surgery are not present, we have to stratify patients benefiting from early surgical intervention and those not profiting from surgery based on their physical status. According to Vollmer et al. [6], the use of the American Society of Anaesthesiologists (ASA) physical status classification is a good option because of its simplicity and ability to stratify patients into low-risk (ASA I-II) and high-risk (III, IV, V) groups with low-risk group patients generally being recommended early cholecystectomy. High-risk group patients are offered nonsurgical therapy, although in case of disease progression and ineffective initial therapy the surgical intervention may be reevaluated [6].

In the group of low-risk patients, the cholecystectomy should be performed as early as possible during the hospitalisation optimally in the first 72 h from the onset of symptoms as it is presumed that the local inflammation worsens with time [6]. Although current Tokyo guidelines as well as World Society of Emergency Surgery guidelines recommend early laparoscopic cholecystectomy also in patients after 72 h, as it is deemed safe because some patients present to hospital already after 72 h from the symptom onset [6]. Patients who have symptoms for longer than 10 days should be planned for delayed cholecystectomy after 6–8 weeks after resolution of the inflammation [6].

In the group of high-risk patients, the initial treatment starts with non-surgical approaches; however, when the disease progresses into gallbladder gangrene/necrosis or perforation or does not respond either to medical therapy or to drainage intervention, the emergency cholecystectomy may be the only option despite the dangers of the surgery [6]. High-risk patients, who handle the acute phase, may be reassessed for delayed surgical intervention and in case of improved physical status may undergo surgery [6]. If the patient's physical status does not improve even after the resolution of the inflammation, these patients are eligible for nonsurgical treatment of gallstone disease [6].

3.3 Gallstone disease in pregnancy

The higher frequency of gallstones in pregnancy compared to non-pregnant patients is based on the physiological functions of hormones released in higher quantities during the pregnancy [7]. Patients with uncomplicated symptomatic gallstone disease with recurrent biliary colic are indicated to undergo cholecystectomy [7]. Although in near term patients suffering from biliary colic, the surgery may by postpone until postpartum [7]. In such cases, it is recommended to perform surgery at least 6 weeks after delivery, but before 3 months after delivery prevent recurrent attacks of biliary colic [7]. Patients with complicated gallstone disease require complex treatment plans. For the patients with acute cholecystitis, the surgery is a safe indication for the mother and foetus in every trimester [7]. However, increased preterm delivery has been associated with the cholecystectomy in the third trimester in several studies [7].

3.4 Surgical approach towards cholecystectomy

Since the discovery of laparoscopy, this technique has been the mainstay in the surgical approach to gallstone disease regarding uncomplicated gallstone disease as well as complicated acute cholecystitis in low-risk and high-risk groups of patients as well as among pregnant patients unless there is an absolute anaesthetic contraindication [4, 6, 7]. The technical aspects of the laparoscopy in acute cholecystitis may be more demanding on the surgeon's skills; therefore, it is no shame to convert to open cholecystectomy when the surgeon is unable to visualise important anatomical structures with the emphasis on the patient's safety.

4. Patient preparation

The basis for successful and safe cholecystectomy is thorough preoperative preparation with the highest emphasis on the patient's physical status and correct indication for surgical therapy. It is important to assess any patient's comorbidities such as cardiac disease, diabetes mellitus as well as factors potentially complicating cholecystectomy such as previous abdominal surgery in the upper half of the abdomen, inflammation, obesity, and pregnancy.

4.1 Preoperative algorithm

1. Setting a valid indication for surgical therapy based on the patient's clinical status, anamnesis, and paraclinical investigations.

2. Assessment of patient's physical status with his comorbidities resulting in the estimation of ASA level and definition of the patient's fitness for surgery.

3. Assessment of local findings—potential signs of acute cholecystitis, biliary obstruction with the choledocholithiasis, any signs of cholecystoenteric fistula, severe liver diseases such as cirrhosis with portal hypertension, or hepatobiliary malignancy.

4. Assessment of the surgeon's technical skills with adaptation and modification of surgical therapy based on the patient's specific factors.

5. Patient's informed consent with a comprehensive explanation of planned surgery with an explanation of potential complications such as biliary or vascular injuries, the need for conversion from laparoscopic approach to laparotomy, the potential necessity for postoperative ERCP or MRCP.

Eventually, this results in correct indication for surgical or nonsurgical therapy, the timing of the surgery, the type of planned surgery with optimal preoperative preparation (thromboprophylaxis according to Caprini score, antibiotics in indicated cases), and well-informed patient about every step of his procedure with solutions for potential complications [8].

5. Surgical approaches towards gallbladder removal

Cholecystectomy is a common surgical procedure indicated in various gallbladder pathologies. Nowadays, it is one of the most commonly performed abdominal surgeries worldwide [2]. Even though the concepts of safe surgery have been adopted, the iatrogenic injuries to biliary structures are still a worldwide problem. Based on the nationwide databases, the incidence of major biliary duct injuries (BDI) is 0.1% in the case of elective laparoscopic cholecystectomy in comparison with 0.3% in emergency laparoscopic cholecystectomy [9]. Total BDI incidence is 0.4% for elective laparoscopic cholecystectomy compared to 0.8% in emergency laparoscopic cholecystectomy and 0.3% in open cholecystectomy [9]. The ongoing existence of complications in gallbladder surgery even more emphasises the importance of the safe surgery concept.

5.1 Open cholecystectomy

The open cholecystectomy (OC) is currently performed in cases of gallbladder cancer, Mirizzi's syndrome, choledochal cyst, and in cases of sclerotising cholangitis. The incision with its localisation must be adequate for good exploration including the use of intraoperative ultrasonography or radical procedure for cancer.

It is important to emphasise that the conversion from laparoscopic approach to open cholecystectomy is not a surgeon's failure. It seems that the risk is higher in men, patients >60 years old, obese patients, patients with cirrhosis, patients after abdominal surgery in the upper part of the abdomen, patients with severe comorbidities, in case of large gallstones, febrilities, gangrenous cholecystitis, the duration of symptoms >48 h in urgent setting [10]. For the patient's safety, the conversion may be considered in case of the surgeon's inability to perform safe complicated laparoscopic cholecystectomy [10]. However, there is no evidence that the conversion will reduce or avert the risk of biliary duct injury [11]. Conversion to open surgery is an option in any difficult case. The most important focus in a cholecystectomy is the safe removal of the gallbladder and the avoidance of bile duct injuries.

5.2 Laparoscopic cholecystectomy

Nowadays, the state-of-the-art surgical therapy for gallstones is laparoscopic cholecystectomy. Laparoscopy is associated with lower postoperative pain, shorter hospital stay, and shorter recovery period [12]. From the first laparoscopic cholecystectomy in the beginning of the 1990s, this technique has changed the therapy for many gallbladder pathologies. Laparoscopic cholecystectomy is indicated for the therapy of acute and chronic cholecystitis, symptomatic gallstone disease, biliary dyskinesis, acalculous cholecystitis, benign gallbladder tumors. According to a recently published meta-analysis, laparoscopic cholecystectomy is also a safe alternative to open cholecystectomy for early gallbladder cancer (stage Tis—T3) with comparable overall survival and the rate of complications [13].

5.2.1 Technique

Initially, we start with the insufflation of the carbon dioxide into the abdominal cavity until we reach the pneumoperitoneum with the intra-abdominal pressure of 15 mmHg. In conventional laparoscopic cholecystectomy, we continue with the placement of the multiple ports depending on the surgeon's experience and skills. Surgeon standardly chooses 3 or 4 ports localised supraumbilically (10 mm port), subxiphoidally (10 mm port), and 1–2 ports in the right subcostal region (5 mm port). The key step in the safe gallbladder removal is the achievement of the critical view of safety (more on the topic in part 6) through meticulous preparation and dissection if this can be achieved. Only in this case, the surgeon can continue with the certainty that he/she has identified the cystic artery and the cystic duct. Both structures are then ligated and interrupted. Later on, we continue with the separation of the gallbladder from the gallbladder bed with the use of electrocautery or the harmonic scalpel. To achieve complete haemostasis, some authors recommend lowering intra-abdominal pressure to 8 mmHg for 2 min to spot potential venous bleeding, which can be undetectable with the intra-abdominal pressure of 15 mmHg. The gallbladder is extracted in the retrieval bag. The drainage in the subhepatic region after uncomplicated cholecystectomy is not routinely recommended. In the end, the trocars should be extracted under direct visualisation, and to prevent incisional hernias, some authors recommend fascial sutures in case of ports larger than 5 mm.

5.2.2 Single-incision laparoscopic cholecystectomy (SILC)

Even though the benefits of the conventional multiple ports access laparoscopic cholecystectomy are undeniable, the efforts to further minimise the traumatisation of the abdominal wall continued with the effort to reduce the number of ports. It was shown that laparoscopic cholecystectomy with the use of only one incision is possible in the clinical setting [14]. The limitations of this technique are the difficulties with the triangulation while using linear laparoscopic tools, limited view, and the possibility of the tools' collisions. SILC can be indicated in patients with uncomplicated disease, with BMI <35 kg/m^2, in whom there is a low probability of conversion either to multiple ports access laparoscopy or open cholecystectomy [15]. However, the role of the SILC compared to conventional LC in day-to-day praxis is debatable based on non-existent clear benefits beyond lower postoperative pain and improved cosmetic effects with no option to clarify the impact on the quality of life [15]. On the other hand, among the disadvantages are the higher occurrence of adverse events with prolonged duration of the surgery and frequent demand for additional port [15].

5.2.3 Common issues in laparoscopic cholecystectomy

The first thing that may compromise our ability to perform safe laparoscopic cholecystectomy may be the problem with the port placement. When we place a supraumbilical port in obese or tall patients in the umbilicus, it can create too low of a view [16]. Another issue with the limitations of fine motor movements may arise when placing the subxiphoidal port too low or not perpendicular to the abdominal wall while creating a form of "port tension" [16]. Tool collisions may happen when we place the surgeon's left-hand port in line with the camera view or the lateral retraction port [16].

The dissection of the gallbladder should be done with the proper incision of the peritoneum, therefore releasing the gallbladder from the liver [16]. A common issue may be with insufficient retraction of the infundibulum inferiorly and laterally and endangering the common hepatic duct or common bile duct by the possibility of an alignment with the cystic duct in the same plane [16]. Important to remember is to use the clips, ligations, or electrosurgical energy on ductal structures only after the visualisation of the regional anatomy [16]. The critical view of safety cannot be achieved unless the bottom third of the cystic plate is fully exposed with adequate dissection of the hepatocystic triangle and clear identification of the cystic duct and the cystic artery [16]. When the CVS is not achievable, the attempt to perform total cholecystectomy is a risk for the patient and we must utilise a bail-out manoeuver [16].

5.3 Robot-assisted cholecystectomy

With the introduction of a robot-assisted surgical system, minimally invasive surgery comes to a new era. In 1998, Himpens first reported the robot-assisted cholecystectomy [17]. Since then, the application of the robotic system has been significantly improved, not only for hepatobiliary and pancreatic surgery but also for urological surgery, gynecology, thoracic surgery, and cardiac surgery. The application of daVinci™ robot-assisted surgical platform overcomes the shortcomings of many laparoscopic techniques [17].

5.3.1 Single-incision robotic cholecystectomy (SIRC)

Robot-assisted surgical platform with the single incision has overcome many limitations of single-incision laparoscopic cholecystectomy with bridling the triangulation, quality of view, and movement options [18]. The indication for SIRC is very similar to that of conventional LC. The relative contraindication being the same for SIRC and SILC; however thanks to better triangulation and surgical skills with the robotic platform, SIRC is being more frequently used in patients with higher BMI, acute cholecystitis, and patients with previous abdominal surgeries in the upper abdomen [19].

6. Concept of safe cholecystectomy

Over the years, there have been many methods for reducing the risk of biliary structures injuries while performing cholecystectomy. Fisher's method, in which the surgeon removes the gallbladder from the gallbladder bed and then identifies the cystic artery and cystic duct which are sequentially ligated, is deemed overcome due to 95% penetration of laparoscopy in the gallbladder surgery [12]. The introduction of the Strassberg method in 1995 meant firstly the preparation of cystic artery and cystic duct in a hepatocystic triangle with identification of cystic duct entering the gallbladder infundibulum [20]. This method is currently called the critical view of safety technique (**Figure 4**) [20].

6.1 Critical view of safety

Critical view of safety (CVS) technique is composed of three steps:

1. Identification and visualisation of hepatocystic triangle without the exposition of the common hepatic duct.

2. Visualisation of infundibular part of the gallbladder with the preparation and separation from gallbladder bed (anterior and posterior view).

3. Visualisation of only 2 structures entering the gallbladder before ligation—a cystic artery and cystic duct [21].

This concept is widely accepted and represents the basis of the safe cholecystectomy model to minimise the incidence of iatrogenic biliary ducts injuries [20].

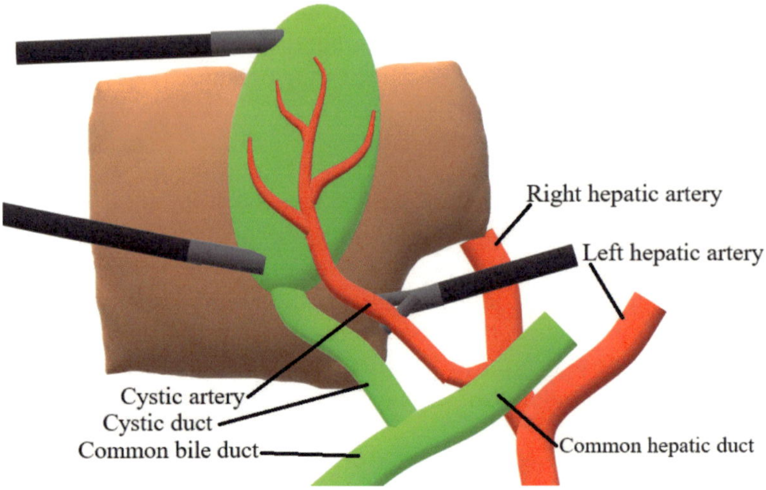

Figure 4.
Schematic image of critical view of safety.

Combination of this method and correct indication for surgery, good preoperative preparation and planning, and meticulous dissection constitute a modern approach towards safe cholecystectomy with reduced risk of biliary structure injury. Due to the scientific verification of reduction in BDIs, the critical view of safety is routinely recommended over other methods [22]. However, CVS cannot always be easily achieved with the most frequent incompleteness in the separation of the infundibular part of the gallbladder from the gallbladder bed. In other cases, the CVS cannot be utilised because of advanced inflammation or scar formation in the hepatocystic triangle due to ongoing or former inflammatory processes [23]. The literature recognised the BDIs to be more frequent in surgeries performed by young residents during the early part of their learning curve in the laparoscopic cholecystectomy. Therefore, it is important for the resident to complete a critical view of safety with the mentoring surgeon to confirm it before ligating any structures [23].

6.2 Bail-out procedures

The concept of CVS cannot be achieved in every case of cholecystectomy; therefore in those situations, the surgeon shall use alternative methods for safe gallbladder removal—the bail-out manoeuver or another method for cystic duct identification. In the setting of acute cholecystitis, the alternative method "fundus-first" has a lower conversion rate and a lower percentage of iatrogenic injuries to the biliary tree [24]. The technique of subtotal cholecystectomy is used as a safe method with minimal risk of injury to the vascular or biliary structures with low conversion volume due to the resection border being out of the risk zone [10]. However, this method has higher amounts of surgical site infections, re-interventions, and rehospitalisations with a longer length of stay [25]. Conversion to open cholecystectomy is an option in difficult cases as well. However, the conversion to OC does not reduce the risk of biliary duct injury as showed in the results of the Belgian multicentre study [26]. In the study of 1089 patients with acute cholecystitis, 116 patients (11.7%) underwent the conversion to open cholecystectomy with the biliary duct injury of 13.7% (16 patients) [26]. Major BDI was present in 6.0% (7 cases) and three cases of the major BDI occurred after the conversion to OC [26]. These results point out the risk of BDI in high-risk patients undergoing cholecystectomy even in cases when the conversion to open gallbladder removal is performed [26].

Therefore, the subtotal cholecystectomy is the preferred choice in surgeons who has low experience with the open cholecystectomy with the exception of large periprocedural haemorrhage, when the method of choice is open cholecystectomy [26]. In the case of complicated cholecystectomy, the intraoperative cholangiography may be a useful method for the identification of anatomical structures and abnormalities with the risk reduction of BDI, although the disadvantage is the need for access to the biliary tree. Another option may be the use of perioperative ultrasonography, which, however, necessitates the need for proper ultrasonography training and knowledge among surgeons.

7. Intraoperative cholangiography and common bile duct exploration

7.1 Intraoperative cholangiography

Intraoperative cholangiography (IOC) can be used intraoperatively for the identification of choledocholithiasis and for visualisation and identification of biliary tree anatomy. The common use of this technique is currently not recommended because of insufficient reduction in complication rate and BDIs during laparoscopic cholecystectomy [27]. The BDIs can appear even in patients in whom the IOC was performed, because of potentially incorrect interpretation of the findings [28]. However, it may be recommended in patients with difficult biliary anatomy and patients, in whom we are unable to perform critical view of safety or there is a perioperative suspicion of a BDI [28]. Importantly, the identification of BDIs with IOC may lead to earlier recognition with a quick therapeutic approach.

Alternatively, the use of indocyanine green fluorescence cholangiography (ICG-C) may be a good option for visualisation of the biliary tree [29]. This method has been suggested by some studies and proved to be effective in acute and chronic gallbladder diseases and in cases, where IOC cannot be used [30].

7.2 Common bile duct exploration

There is an ongoing controversy about an ideal solution for patients with gallstones and bile duct stones. Historically, the method of choice was the open cholecystectomy with the common bile duct exploration (CBDE), which was replaced due to the progress in the laparoscopic and endoscopic methods. With the improvement of the ERCP, the standard of care for patients with cholecystolithiasis and choledocholithiasis became the preoperative ERCP with the endoscopic sphincterotomy and extraction of the choledocholiths with the subsequent laparoscopic cholecystectomy [31]. It is important to say that the open CBDE was the gold standard during the era of the open cholecystectomies for patients in a need of bile duct stones extraction, with the ERCP being used secondarily. The improvements in the laparoscopy lead to a decline in OC and surgeons started to use and rely more on the ERCP to solve the choledocholithiasis. Laparoscopic CBDE is currently an advanced method and in some centres, it is a method of choice. Although some studies have shown the advantages (lower amount of interventions, lower economic burden, shorter length of stay) of the one-stage procedure (LC + laparoscopic CBDE) in comparison with two-stage procedures (pre- or postoperative ERCP + LC), this practice was not generally accepted [32]. Nowadays, the method of choice is two-stage management with the preoperative ERCP and subsequent LC. Even though the ERCP is considered safe, it is a method with high chances of complications with acute post-ERCP pancreatitis being the most common post-ERCP complication with the high economic burden on healthcare systems [33].

Laparoendoscopic rendezvous (LERV) as a combination of laparoscopy and endoscopy is an attractive method in management of patients with cholecystolithiasis and choledocholithiasis. Recent meta-analysis of eight studies compared LERV with two-stage management (preoperative ERCP + LC) in 1061 patients with gallstones and bile duct stones [34]. A total of 542 patients were treated with LERV technique and 519 patients underwent ERCP with subsequent LC. Between the two groups there were no significant differences in the bile duct clearance (OR 2.20, $P = 0.10$), postoperative bleeding (OR 0.67, $P = 0.37$), postoperative cholangitis (OR 0.66, $P = 0.53$), postoperative bile leak (OR 0.87, $P = 0.81$), or conversion to different approaches (OR 0.75, $P = 0.62$) [34]. Total time of surgery was longer in the LERV group ($MD = 44.93$, $P < 0.00001$); however, the advantage of the LERV technique was lower incidence of postoperative pancreatitis (OR 0.26, $P = 0.0003$) and lower overall morbidity (OR 0.41, $P < 0.0001$) with a shorter length of hospital stay ($MD = -3.52$, $P < 0.00001$) [34]. The authors of the meta-analysis concluded the LERV to be equivalent to standard two-stage management of patients with gallstones and bile duct stones [34].

In current practice, there are clear guidelines by the British Society of Gastroenterology recommending the extraction and clearance of the choledocholiths from the CBD [35]. Although, laparoscopic cholecystectomy is a gold standard for gallstone disease, a consensus on the optimal therapeutic approach in the management of bile duct stones has not been reached. Thanks to the improvements in the laparoscopic technique and surgical skills, the single-stage LC + CBDE has shown its benefits and promise. However, the very limitations are based on the necessity of advanced surgical skills with technical demandingness and the availability of the ERCP rule in favour of the two-stage approaches in the majority of centres [36]. The future may lie with the LERV technique, although as a novel therapeutic approach there are still needed further randomised control trials to decide the optimal therapeutic approach for patients with gallstones and bile duct stones.

8. Complications of gallstone surgical therapy

Invasive procedures may be complicated by a number of factors related either to the surgeon and his skillset or patient's characteristics with the clinical findings and anatomical variations. In the case of laparoscopic cholecystectomy, the complications rate varies from 0.5 to 6%:

- Biliary duct injury with the incidence 0.1–0.6%
- Bleeding and vascular injury with the incidence 0.04–1.22%
- Gallbladder perforation 10–30% [37]

Surgeon experience

Incidence of complication is significantly related to the surgeon's experience. Some authors estimated 50 performed laparoscopic cholecystectomies to complete the training in this procedure. However, the end of the learning curve for laparoscopic cholecystectomy is somewhat debatable. Some studies have evaluated the decrease in the bile duct injuries or conversion and complication rates, while others focused on operation time, but the definitive criteria are still being formed [38]. Nonetheless, experienced surgeons have the lowest complication rates; therefore, an increasing number of institutions require proof of fundamental skills in laparoscopic surgery.

Timing of surgery and patients selection

Patients with acute cholecystitis with inflammatory changes have a higher likelihood for a complication during surgery. Also, a higher rate of complications can be expected in patients with chronic cholecystitis with fibrotic changes in the hepatoduodenal ligament and gallbladder fossa. Choledocholithiasis should be revealed before surgery. Patient's history and a series of examinations can refer to the presence of bile duct stones. Performing routine preoperative ERCP is not currently recommended [39]. It is reasonable only in cases of suspicion of common bile duct stones (dilatation of common bile ducts, clinical or laboratory picture of pancreatitis, fever, elevated inflammatory markers, jaundice).

8.1 Biliary duct injury

Clinical manifestation of biliary duct injury (BDI) can be various and it depends on the kind of injury. BDI can run asymptomatically in cases of small damages to the biliary tree to acute process in cases of transection or occlusion of the common bile duct. Approximately only 25% of cases of BDI are recognised during laparoscopy and the detailed description of the case is very important [40].

Type A—This group represents leakage from the gallbladder bed, minor hepatic ducts, and cystic duct without damage to the biliary tree (**Figure 5**).

Type B—Occlusion of the aberrant right hepatic duct (**Figure 6**).

Type C—Transection of the aberrant right hepatic duct (**Figure 7**).

Cystic dust drainage into an aberrant right hepatic duct is a variation seen in approximately 2% of patients. Injuries type B and C are usually caused by confusion of the aberrant right hepatic duct with the cystic duct. Patients with type B injury may remain asymptomatic for a long period of time. Right upper quadrant pain, fever, elevated liver enzymes, and markers of inflammation can be signs of cholangitis, and ultrasonography (US) will show dilatation of the right part of the biliary tree. The occlusion leads to dilatation of the right part of the biliary tree, fibrotic changes, and finally to lobar atrophy. Type C injury causes biliary leakage.

Type D—This group of injuries represents mural lesions of the common bile duct without interruption of its course (**Figure 8**). The result of this damage is a biliary leakage and it can progress to a more serious type E injury.

Type E—This injuries involve interruptions of the extrahepatic biliary ducts and depending on the location of the injury, they are divided into five subgroups (Bismuth classification) [39].

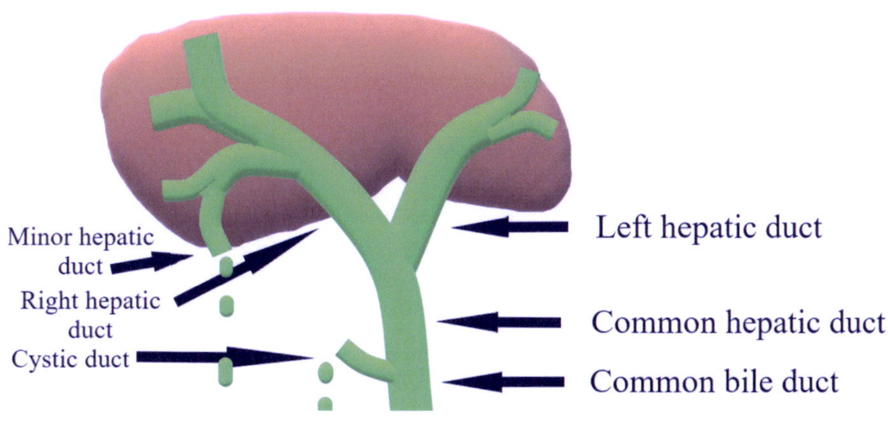

Figure 5.
Schematic image of leakage from the gallbladder bed, minor hepatic ducts, and cystic duct without damage to the biliary tree (Type A).

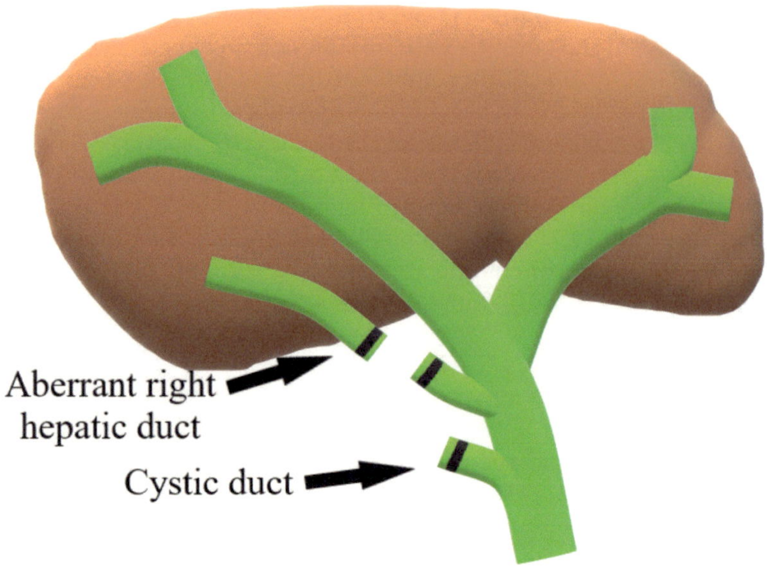

Figure 6.
Schematic image of occluded aberrant right hepatic duct (Type B).

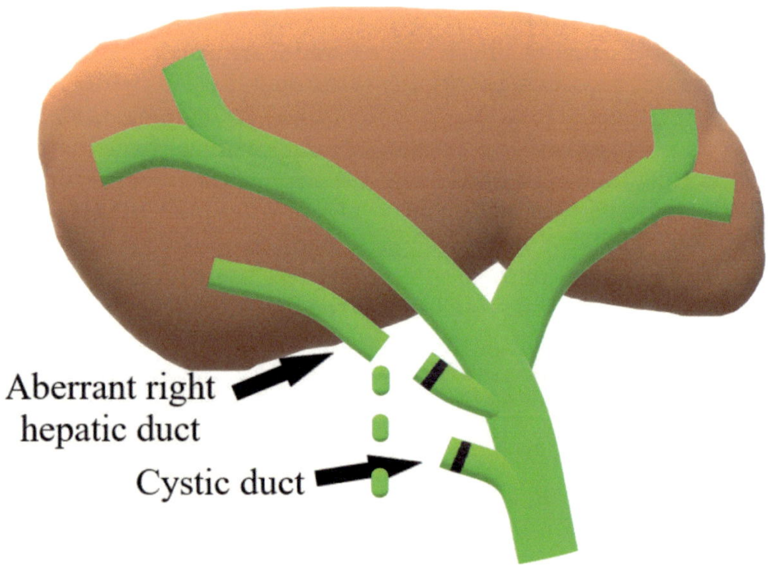

Figure 7.
Schematic image of transected aberrant right hepatic duct (Type C).

E1—(Bismuth Type I)—transection more than 2 cm from the confluence of the right and left hepatic ducts (**Figure 9**).

E2—(Bismuth Type II)—transection less than 2 cm from the confluence (**Figure 10**).

E3—(Bismuth Type III)—transection in the confluence (**Figure 11**).

E4—(Bismuth Type IV)— separation of major duct from the right and left hepatic duct (**Figure 12**).

E5—(Bismuth Type V)—Interruption of the aberrant right hepatic duct (Type C) combined with the injury in the hilum (**Figure 13**).

DOI: http://dx.doi.org/10.5772/intechopen.100570

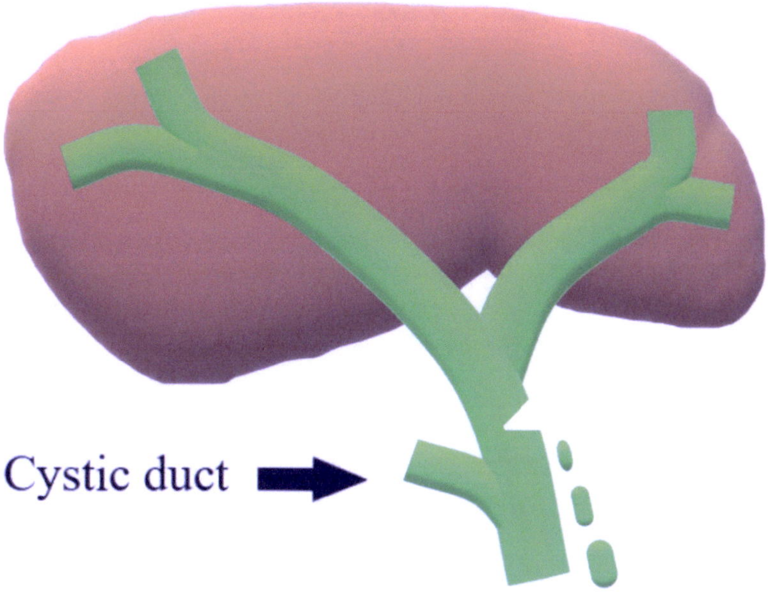

Figure 8.
Schematic image of lesion to the common bile duct without interruption of its course (Type D).

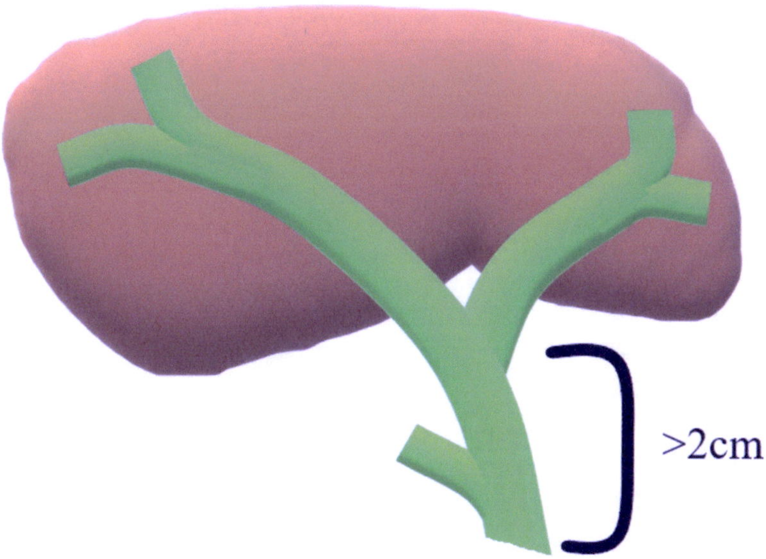

Figure 9.
Schematic image of transected CHD (Type E, Bismuth Type I).

Bismuth classification of BDI was the first scheme published in 1982 [41]. After this classification, other more complex classification systems were proposed. For clinical use, BDI are usually divided into two groups: minor and major injuries.

8.1.1 Diagnosis of biliary injury

Minor BDI are associated with partial lesions without tissue and continuity loss. Major BDI are associated with tissue loss or interruption or occlusion of the main hepatic duct. In a situation when BDI is recognised during laparoscopic surgery,

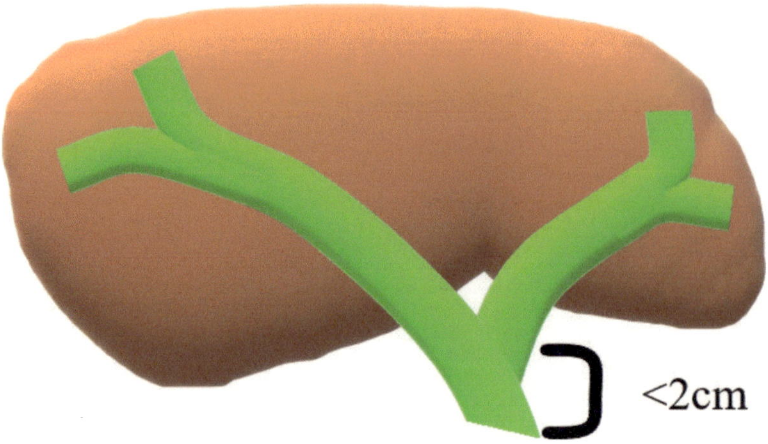

Figure 10.
Schematic image of transected CHD (Type E, Bismuth Type II).

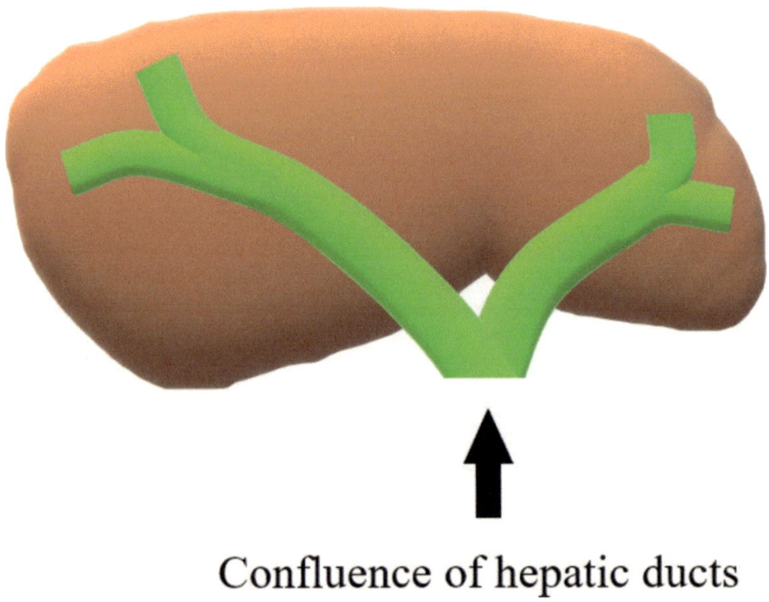

Figure 11.
Schematic image of transected CHD in the confluence (Type E, Bismuth Type III).

conversion to an open procedure and attempt for a repair is recommended only when the surgeon is skilled in advanced biliary surgery. Non-expert immediate attempts for repair are associated with worse outcomes, and they can compromise later revisions; therefore, an intraoperative consultation of an expert is recommended and patients especially with major BDI should be referred to a hepatobiliary centres with multidisciplinary care [39, 41]. External drainage of the subhepatic space is recommended, and a patient should be referred to the centre early because delayed transfers are associated with a higher rate of complications [42].

In case of intraoperative suspicion of BDI or when patients' biliary anatomy is unclear, intraoperative cholangiography may be helpful [28]. Currently, it is not generally recommended to perform routine intraoperative cholangiography because it is not associated with a significant reduction of BDI rates and it can lead to BDI itself because of misinterpretation of patients' anatomy.

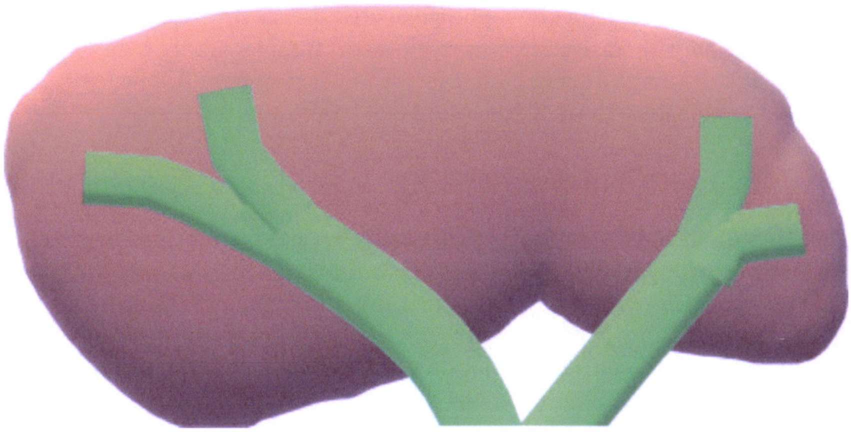

Figure 12.
Schematic image of separated major duct from the right and left hepatic duct (Type E, Bismuth Type IV).

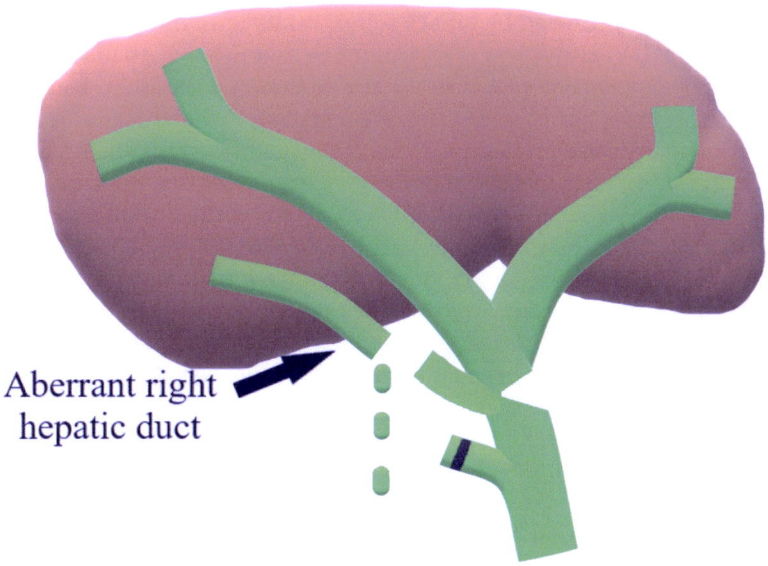

Figure 13.
Schematic image of interrupted aberrant right hepatic duct (Type C) combined with the injury in the hilum (Type E, Bismuth Type V).

8.2 Bile leaks

This group represents biliary injuries types A, C, D, and E.

Type A leak is localised from the cystic duct or the bile duct Luschka [43]. It can be caused by loosen ligature or dislodged clips because of a frail tissue or obstruction of the cystic duct remnant.

Bile duct of Luschka is a minor accessory bile duct that directly enters the gallbladder in the bed. Clinically, significant leakage from the duct after cholecystectomy is not very common.

Types C and D leaks are related to BDI to aberrant and main ducts.

Clinical presentation depends on the extent of the lesion. Minor lesions with small perihepatic collections may remain asymptomatic for a long time or may resolve spontaneously. Major lesions are followed by massive biliary leakage and affected patients are usually symptomatic. Typical symptoms are abdominal pain, bilious collections or bilious ascites, fever. In this case, jaundice is a variable sign because the serum level of bilirubin can be just slightly elevated. Leucocytosis and elevated serum levels of alkaline phosphatase and gamma-glutamyl transferase are common [39].

If subhepatic drainage during cholecystectomy is performed, bile leakage is usually obvious and the extent of the lesion can be indirectly estimated.

8.2.1 Radiologic examinations and management

Transabdominal ultrasonography (US) is the basic examination that can describe perihepatic fluid collections and the biliary tree diameter. If the US finding is unclear and the symptomatology is worsening, the CT may be helpful to detect free intraperitoneal fluid or associated vascular injury (triphasic CT) [44].

Large collections or free peritoneal fluid of larger volume can be percutaneously drained and examined for assessment of bilirubin levels. It is recommended to take a sample for microbiological examination and in case of clinical and laboratory proof of sepsis development (elevated inflammatory markers), empiric antibiotic treatment is reasonable, particularly in patients with a history of biliary infections and preoperative ERCP and stenting [44].

Bile leakage can be verified by biliary scintigraphy with hepatobiliary iminodiacetic acid scan (HIDA). It is very sensitive in the diagnosis of an ongoing bile leak, though it cannot anatomically localise the site of the leakage. Major leaks can be obvious on early scans, but if early scans are negative, delayed scans after 3 h from tracer injection are recommended [45].

MRCP is a non-invasive method that can be used for the diagnosis of bile leak and localisation of the leak site. It is particularly important in the case of hilar injury [46].

ERCP is an examination that can determine the side of the BDI and offers a possibility of the insertion of the biliary stents. Stenting across the ampulla can solve the majority of BDI types A and D and reduce the pressure in the biliary tree [39]. Sphincterotomy may be performed without stenting; however, it is recommended in cases of biliary obstruction because of choledocholithiasis [39].

In cases when a minimally invasive approach does not solve patients' state, if there is biliary peritonitis and evidence of progressive sepsis, an operative exploration and washout are recommended [44].

In type A injuries, stents can be removed endoscopically usually after 2 weeks if there is no ongoing biliary leak on ERCP [39]. In types C and D injuries, repeated HIDA scans are recommended after 2–4 weeks after stent insertion and stents can be removed if there is no leak on a follow-up ERCP [39]. If the leak persists, stents can be replaced or sphincterotomy can be performed to facilitate the bile flow [39]. Patients with type D injuries require close follow-up due to stricture development or progression to type E injuries in case of larger defects of the biliary wall [39]. Also, endoscopic treatment is less effective in the type C injuries because the aberrant right hepatic duct is disconnected from the proximal part of the biliary tree [39].

Occlusive BDI of the right hepatic bile duct usually leads to segmental cholestasis, fibrosis, and right lobar atrophy. It can be asymptomatic but some patients can suffer from cholangitis or hepaticolithiasis. US and CT may show dilatated duct of the right part of the liver with focal atrophy of the liver tissue. ERCP and MRCP will show the site of the obstruction of the right hepatic duct. The treatment of this BDI is surgical. In case when fibrosis and atrophy are not advanced, a hepaticojejunostomy should be performed. Significant atrophy may require resection.

8.2.2 Transections of common hepatic duct

Type E injuries are localised at the common hepatic duct and are the most serious. Transections of the common hepatic duct are usually recognised at the time of surgery, because of a biliary leak. If there is only a limited mural lesion of the common bile duct, placing a T-tube drain could be a solution. Primary repair attempts should be avoided, especially in case of normal diameter of the common hepatic duct and tissue loss because the probability for breakdown is high and it can lead to bile duct strictures during the healing process [44]. These attempts, especially if they are performed by an inexperienced surgeon, can make the future revisions more difficult [44]. Significant damage of the common hepatic duct is preferably solved by hepaticojejunostomy [44].

Clinical symptoms depend on the nature of an injury. Occlusive injuries lead to jaundice development and elevated liver function tests. Radiological examinations will show diffuse dilatation of intrahepatic bile ducts, and ERCP will verify complete obstruction of the common hepatic duct. In order to decompress the intrahepatic bile ducts, percutaneous transhepatic drainage (PTD) and percutaneous transhepatic cholangiography (PTC) should be performed. Both liver lobes have to be drained and it can require placing percutaneous drains to both intrahepatic parts of the biliary tree. In cases of strictures due to inappropriately placed clips or ligatures, ERCP with the dilatation and stent insertion may be helpful. Endoscopic treatment is not very effective in cases of complete occlusion and if the length of the stricture is longer than 1 cm. The treatment of choice is surgery and hepaticojejunostomy Roux-en Y [44, 47].

8.3 Bleeding and vascular injury

Bleeding from the gallbladder bed is not a rare complication, especially in cases of fibrotic changes in chronic cholecystitis. If laparoscopic attempts for bleeding control fail, it usually requires immediate conversion and ligation [48].

Arterial bleeding is usually caused by the cystic artery transection and can be controlled by clipping, but a surgeon must avoid injury to the right hepatic artery. Injuries of the right hepatic artery require a high level of technical expertise, and the efficiency of reconstruction is questionable. Many right hepatic artery injuries remain unrecognised because its interruption is usually well tolerated [44].

Bleeding from trocar sites should be avoided with direct visualisation after removal.

8.4 Bowel injuries

Bowel injuries are a rare complication. If the bowel injury is recognised intraoperatively, it must be unconditionally repaired. Unspotted bowel injuries may lead to sepsis development after the procedure and require broad-spectrum antibiotic treatment and laparotomy for reparation. Clinical symptoms involve abdominal pain, hypotension with tachycardia with the laboratory picture of leucocytosis or leucopenia, and elevated serum inflammatory markers. In cases when clinical symptoms are mild, a patient does not develop sepsis and an adequate drainage can be achieved, management can be continued as for controlled entercutaneous fistulas [39].

9. Conclusion

Nowadays, the laparoscopic cholecystectomy is the state-of-the-art surgical therapy for gallstones disease. The primary concept is the safety of the patient; therefore, the surgeon must be aware of the anatomy variations and has to be prepared to react to them. The first thing young residents have to learn is the technique of critical view of safety to reduce the risk of biliary duct injuries. Although we may do every effort to minimise the risks of complications, those will happen nonetheless. Therefore, every surgeon has to be aware of the basics in the management of cholecystectomy complications.

Conflict of interest

The authors declare no conflict of interest.

Author details

Peter Dubovan, Ramadan Aziri and Miroslav Tomáš*
Department of Surgical Oncology, National Cancer Institute in Bratislava, Slovak Medical University, Bratislava, Slovak Republic

*Address all correspondence to: dr.mirotomas@gmail.com

References

[1] Yannos S, Athanasios P. History of biliary surgery. World Journal of Surgery. 2013;**37**(5):1006-1012. DOI: 10.1007/s00268-013-1960-6

[2] Eurostat. Surgical Operations and Procedures Statistics [Internet]. 2020. Available from: https://ec.europa.eu/eurostat/statistics-explained/index.php?title=Surgical_operations_and_procedures_statistics#Number_of_surgical_operations_and_procedures [Accessed: 08 June 2021]

[3] Skandalakis JE, Colborn GL, Weidman TA, et al. Skandalakis' Surgical Anatomy. 1st ed. Broken Hill. PMP; 2004. p. 1720. ISBN-10: 9789603990741

[4] Uptodate [Internet]. Wolters Kluwer Inc. UpToDate: The Clinical Answers You Need—Anytime, Anywhere [Updated: 01 September 2020; cited: 05 July 2021]. Approach to the Management of Gallstones. Available from: https://www.uptodate.com/contents/approach-to-the-management-of-gallstones?topicRef=3685&source=see_link Subscription required

[5] Uptodate [Internet]. Wolters Kluwer Inc. UpToDate: The Clinical Answers You Need—Anytime, Anywhere [Updated: 21 May 2021; cited: 05 July 2021]. Gallbladder Cancer: Epidemiology, Risk Factors, Clinical Features, and Diagnosis. Available from: https://www.uptodate.com/contents/gallbladder-cancer-epidemiology-risk-factors-clinical-features-and-diagnosis?topicRef=673&source=see_link. Subscription required

[6] Uptodate [Internet]. Wolters Kluwer Inc. UpToDate: The Clinical Answers You Need—Anytime, Anywhere [Updated: 22 December 2020; cited 05 July 2021]. Treatment of Acute Calculous Cholecystitis. Available from: https://www.uptodate.com/contents/treatment-of-acute-calculous-cholecystitis?topicRef=3685&source=see_link#H3556800859. Subscription required

[7] Uptodate [Internet]. Wolters Kluwer Inc. UpToDate: The Clinical Answers You Need—Anytime, Anywhere [Updated: 17 June 2021; cited: 05 July 2021]. Gallstone Diseases in Pregnancy. Available from: https://www.uptodate.com/contents/gallstone-diseases-in-pregnancy?topicRef=3684&source=see_link#H210627438. Subscription required

[8] Cronin M, Dengler N, Krauss ES, et al. Completion of the updated caprini risk assessment model (2013 version). Clinical and Applied Thrombosis/Hemostasis. 2019;**2019**:25. DOI: 10.1177/1076029619838052

[9] Kapoor VK. Epidemiology of bile duct injury. In: Kapoor V, editor. Postcholecystectomy Bile Duct Injury. Singapore: Springer; 2020. pp. 109-125

[10] Strasberg S, Pucci MJ, Brunt LM, et al. Subtotal cholecystectomy—"Fenestrating" vs "Reconstituting" subtypes and the prevention of bile duct injury: Definition of the optimal procedure in difficult operative conditions. Journal of the American College of Surgeons. 2016;**222**(1):89-96

[11] Altieri MS, Yang J, Obeid N, Zhu C, et al. Bile duct injury and decreasing utilization of intraoperative cholangiogram and common bile duct exploration over 14 years: An analysis of outcomes in New York State. Surgical Endoscopy. 2017;**32**(2):667-674

[12] Keus F, de Jong JA, Gooszen HG, et al. Laparoscopic versus open cholecystectomy for patients with symptomatic cholecystolithiasis. Cochrane Database of Systematic Reviews. 2006;**4**:CD006231

[13] Feng X, Cao JS, Chen MY, et al. Laparoscopic surgery for early gallbladder carcinoma: A systematic review and meta-analysis. World Journal of Clinical Cases. 2020;**8**(6): 1074-1086. DOI: 10.12998/wjcc.v8.i6.1074

[14] Pisanu A, Reccia I, Porceddu G, et al. Meta-analysis of prospective randomized studies comparing single-incision laparoscopic cholecystectomy (SILC) and conventional multiport laparoscopic cholecystectomy (CMLC). Journal of Gastrointestinal Surgery. 2012;**16**(9):1790-1801

[15] Evers L, Bouvy N, Branje D, et al. Single-incision laparoscopic cholecystectomy versus conventional four-port laparoscopic cholecystectomy: A systematic review and meta-analysis. Surgical Endoscopy. 2017;**31**(9):3437-3448

[16] Asbun HJ, Shah MM, Ceppa EP, et al. The SAGES Manual of Biliary Surgery. Cham, Switzerland: Springer; 2020

[17] Himpens J, Leman G, Cadiere GB. Telesurgical laparoscopic cholecystectomy. Surgical Endoscopy. 1998;**12**(8):1091

[18] Gonzalez A, Murcia CH, Romero R, et al. A multicenter study of initial experience with single-incision robotic cholecystectomies (SIRC) demonstrating a high success rate in 465 cases. Surgical Endoscopy. 2016;**30**(7):2951-2960

[19] Escobar-Dominguez JE, Hernandez-Murcia C, Gonzalez AM. Description of robotic single site cholecystectomy and a review of outcomes. Journal of Surgical Oncology. 2015;**112**(3):284-288

[20] Strasberg SM, Hertl M, Soper NJ. An analysis of the problem of biliary injury during laparoscopic cholecystectomy. Journal of the American College of Surgeons. 1995;**180**(1):101-125

[21] Strasberg SM, Brunt LM. Rationale and use of the critical view of safety in laparoscopic cholecystectomy. Journal of the American College of Surgeons. 2010;**211**(1):132-138

[22] Sgaramella LI, Gurrado A, Pasculli A, et al. The critical view of safety during laparoscopic cholecystectomy: Strasberg Yes or No? An Italian multicentre study. Surgical Endoscopy. 2020;**35**(7):3698-3708

[23] Strasberg SM. A three-step conceptual roadmap for avoiding bile duct injury in laparoscopic cholecystectomy: An invited perspective review. Journal of Hepato-Biliary-Pancreatic Sciences. 2019;**26**(4):123-127. DOI: 10.1002/jhbp.616

[24] Strasberg SM, Gouma DJ. 'Extreme' vasculobiliary injuries: Association with fundus-down cholecystectomy in severely inflamed gallbladders. HPB (Oxford). 2012;**14**:1-8

[25] Lidsky ME, Speicher PJ, Ezekian B, et al. Subtotal cholecystectomy for the hostile gallbladder: Failure to control the cystic duct results in significant morbidity. HPB: The Official Journal of the International Hepato Pancreato Biliary Association. 2017;**19**:547-545

[26] Navez B, Ungureanu F, Michiels M, et al. Surgical management of acute cholecystitis: Results of a 2-year prospective multicenter survey in Belgium. Surgical Endoscopy. 2012;**26**(9):2436-2445

[27] Ding GQ, Cai W, Qin MF. Is intraoperative cholangiography necessary during laparoscopic cholecystectomy for cholelithiasis? World Journal of Gastroenterology. 2015;**1**(7):2147-2151

[28] Brunt LM, Deziel DJ, Telem DA, et al. Safe cholecystectomy multi-society practice guideline and state of the art consensus conference on

prevention of bile duct injury during cholecystectomy. Annals of Surgery. 2020;**272**(1):3-23

[29] Goldstein SD, Lautz TB. Fluorescent cholangiography during laparoscopic cholecystectomy: Shedding new light on biliary anatomy. JAMA Surgery. 2020; **155**(10):978

[30] Pesce A, Piccolo G, La Greca G, Puleo S. Utility of fluorescent cholangiography during laparoscopic cholecystectomy: A systematic review. World Journal of Gastroenterology. 2015;**21**(25):7877-7883

[31] Prasson P, Bai X, Zhang Q, Liang T. One-stage laproendoscopic procedure versus two-stage procedure in the management for gallstone disease and biliary duct calculi: A systemic review and meta-analysis. Surgical Endoscopy. 2016;**30**:3582-3590

[32] Bansal VK et al. Single-stage laparoscopic common bile duct exploration and cholecystectomy versus two-stage endoscopic stone extraction followed by laparoscopic cholecystectomy for patients with concomitant gallbladder stones and common bile duct stones: A randomized controlled trial. Surgical Endoscopy. 2014;**28**(3):875-885

[33] Luo H, Zhao L, Leung J, et al. Routine pre-procedural rectal indometacin versus selective post-procedural rectal indometacin to prevent pancreatitis in patients undergoing endoscopic retrograde cholangiopancreatography: A multicentre, single-blinded, randomised controlled trial. Lancet. 2016;**387**: 2293-2301

[34] Lin Y, Su Y, Yan J, et al. Laparoendoscopic rendezvous versus ERCP followed by laparoscopic cholecystectomy in the management of cholecystocholedocholithiasis: A systemic review and meta-analysis. Surgical Endoscopy. 2020;**34**(9): 4214-4224

[35] Williams E, Beckingham I, El Sayed G, et al. Updated guideline on the management of common bile duct stones (CBDS). Gut. 2017;**66**(5):765-782. DOI: 10.1136/gutjnl-2016-312317. Epub 2017 Jan 25

[36] Wandling MW, Hungness ES, Pavey ES, et al. Nationwide assessment of trends in choledocholithiasis management in the United States from 1998 to 2013. JAMA Surgery. 2016; **151**(12):1125-1130. DOI: 10.1001/jamasurg.2016.2059

[37] Radunovic M, Lazovic R, Popovic N, et al. Complications of laparoscopic cholecystectomy: Our experience from a retrospective analysis. Open Access Macedonian Journal of Medical Sciences. 2016;**4**(4):641-646. DOI: 10.3889/oamjms.2016.128

[38] Reitano E, de'Angelis N, Schembari E, et al. Learning curve for laparoscopic cholecystectomy has not been defined: A systematic review. ANZ Journal of Surgery. 2021;**91**(9): E554-E560. DOI: 10.1111/ans.17021. Epub 2021 Jun 28

[39] Uptodate [Internet]. Wolters Kluwer Inc. UpToDate: The Clinical Answers You Need—Anytime, Anywhere [Updated: 06 February 2020; cited 05 July 2021]. Complications of Laparoscopic Cholecystectomy. Available from: https://www.uptodate.com/contents/complications-of-laparoscopic-cholecystectomy. Subscription required

[40] Stewart L. Iatrogenic biliary injuries: Identification, classification, and management. Surgical Clinics of North America. 2014;**94**(2):297-310. DOI: 10.1 016/j.suc.2014.01.008

[41] Bismuth H, Majno PE. Biliary strictures: Classification based on the principles of surgical treatment. World Journal of Surgery. 2001;**25**(10):1241-1244. DOI: 10.1007/s00268-001-0102-8

[42] Wang X, Yu WL, Fu XH, Zhu B, Zhao T, Zhang YJ. Early versus delayed surgical repair and referral for patients with bile duct injury: A systematic review and meta-analysis. Annals of Surgery. 2020;**271**(3):449-459. DOI: 10.1097/SLA.0000000000003448

[43] Siiki A, Rinta-Kiikka I, Sand J, et al. Biodegradable biliary stent in the endoscopic treatment of cystic duct leak after cholecystectomy: The first case report and review of literature. Journal of Laparoendoscopic & Advanced Surgical Techniques. Part A. 2015;**25**(5): 419-422. DOI: 10.1089/lap.2015.0068

[44] de'Angelis N et al. 2020 WSES guidelines for the detection and management of bile duct injury during cholecystectomy. World Journal of Emergency Surgery. 2021;**16**:30. DOI: 10.1186/s13017-021-00369-w

[45] Snyder E, Kashyap S, Lopez PP. Hepatobiliary iminodiacetic acid scan. In: StatPearls [Internet]. Treasure Island (FL): StatPearls Publishing; 2021

[46] Cieszanowski A, Stadnik A, Lezak A, et al. Detection of active bile leak with Gd-EOB-DTPA enhanced MR cholangiography: Comparison of 20-25 min delayed and 60-180 min delayed images. European Journal of Radiology. 2013;**82**(12):2176-2182. DOI: 10.1016/j.ejrad.2013.08.021. Epub 2013 Aug 23

[47] Shimada H, Endo I, Shimada K, Matsuyama R, Kobayashi N, Kubota K. The current diagnosis and treatment of benign biliary stricture. Surgery Today. 2012;**42**:1143

[48] Schembari E, Bortolussi C, Coco O, et al. Peritoneal lavage: A simple tool to prevent bleeding during and after laparoscopic cholecystectomy. Journal of Blood Medicine. 2019;**10**:279-281. DOI: 10.2147/JBM.S215438. eCollection 2019

Chapter 4

Infections of Biliary Tract

Hema Prakash Kumari Pilli and Vijayalakshmi Payala

Abstract

Biliary tract infections include cholangitis and cholecystitis. They are associated with high morbidity and mortality in elderly patients with comorbid disease. The most common infecting organisms are Enterobacteriaceae ascending from the gastrointestinal tract, Gram-positive pathogens like Enterococci spp.; the infections are rarely caused by fungi, viruses, and parasites. The prime reason for biliary tract infections is the ascending infection due to the reflux of duodenal contents and also the blood-borne infection or infection spreading through the portal-venous channels. The other predisposing conditions causing biliary tract infections include critical illnesses such as trauma, burns, sepsis, HIV infection, immunosuppression, diabetes, non-biliary surgery, and childbirth. The infection is reduced by β-lactam antibiotics or their derivatives, cephalosporins, carbapenems, fluoroquinolones, etc. Empiric treatment with piperacillin/tazobactam or a cephalosporin with or without metronidazole is recommended for moderate and severe acute cholecystitis irrespective of whether there is growth by culture. Patients with severe cholecystitis are unfortunately difficult to identify properly, both clinically and radiologically, because clinical symptoms are unexpected, and imaging investigations are frequently ambiguous. However, there are significant differences in morbidity and death rates between individuals with mild cholecystitis and those with severe cholecystitis. Preventing related consequences requires early identification and effective therapy of individuals at risk of severe cholecystitis.

Keywords: acute cholecystitis, bacteria, chronic cholecystitis, antibiotics, cholangitis

1. Introduction

Biliary tract infections, such as biliary colic, cholangitis, cholecystitis, and cholelithiasis, are the most commonly encountered health disorders globally as a result of bile duct obstruction. Gallstones are relatively prevalent in the United States and many other industrialized countries, and they are usually asymptomatic. Gallstones are projected to affect 25 million adults in the United States (Everhart et al.) [1]. Bacterial infection of the bile can result in severe morbidity and mortality [Sifri and Madoff] [2]. Bile stasis, inflammation, and the loss of mechanical barriers can all lead to bacterial infection of the bile, which can end in severe morbidity and death. Obstruction is hypothesized to cause increased intraluminal pressure, impaired blood supply and lymphatic drainage, and acute inflammation in the presence of supersaturated bile (Indar and Beckingham) [3]. The pathogenesis of biliary tract infections, the microbial pathogens involved, and antibiotic treatment options are discussed in this article.

IntechOpen

2. Current scenario

Gallstone disease is a substantial health problem in developed countries, according to existing literature. Gallstones are believed to affect 10–15% of the general population, with considerable variations across nations. Gallstone-related problems affect between 20 and 40% of individuals with gallstones, with an annual incidence of 1–3%; acute calculus cholecystitis (ACC) is the first clinical manifestation in 10–15% of cases [4].

3. Anatomy of biliary tract

The gallbladder is a part of the digestive system. The gallbladder is a thin-walled sac with three anatomic parts: the fundus, corpus, and infundibulum [1]. It is normally located between both hepatic lobes. **Figure 1** depicts the gall bladder location in the human body, and **Figure 2** represents the gall bladder anatomy. The gallbladder empties into the cystic duct, a passive conduit with a mucosa comprising spiral valves and with a diameter of about 7 mm in humans (Valves of Heister). This duct has no sphincteric structure and empties into the common bile duct. As it enters the duodenal wall and forms the ampulla of Vater, the common bile duct passes through the head of the pancreas, finishing in the sphincter of Oddi [6].

Approximately, 10% of individuals are estimated to have one or more biliary duct abnormalities; however, not all of them are difficult to identify during surgery. The so-called triple confluence, which is an abnormality defined by simultaneous emptying of the right posterior duct, right anterior duct, and left hepatic duct into the common hepatic duct [Mortele and Ros] [7], is a frequent variation of the major hepatic biliary branching. The right hepatic duct is almost non-existent in individuals with this variation. The right posterior duct and its union with the right anterior or left hepatic duct are two more common anatomic variations of the biliary tree branching.

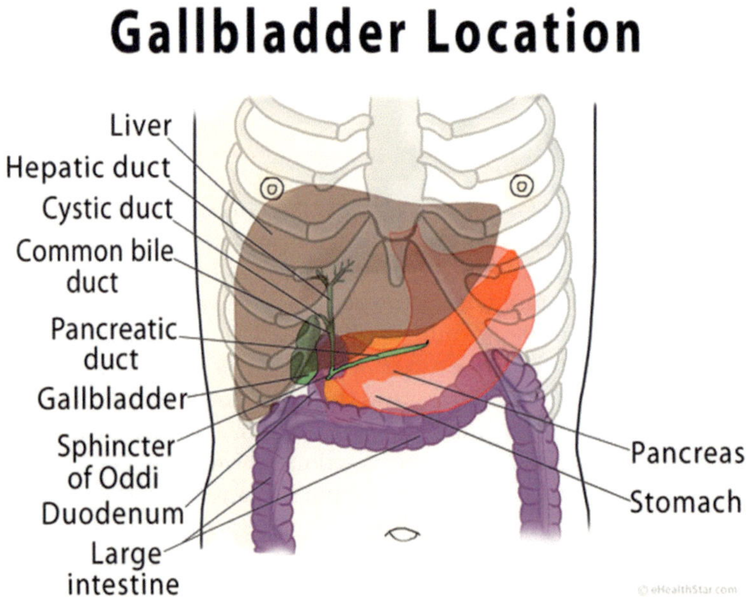

Figure 1.
Gallbladder lies beneath the lower liver edge at the bottom of the rib cage. (Jan Modric, 2017) [5].

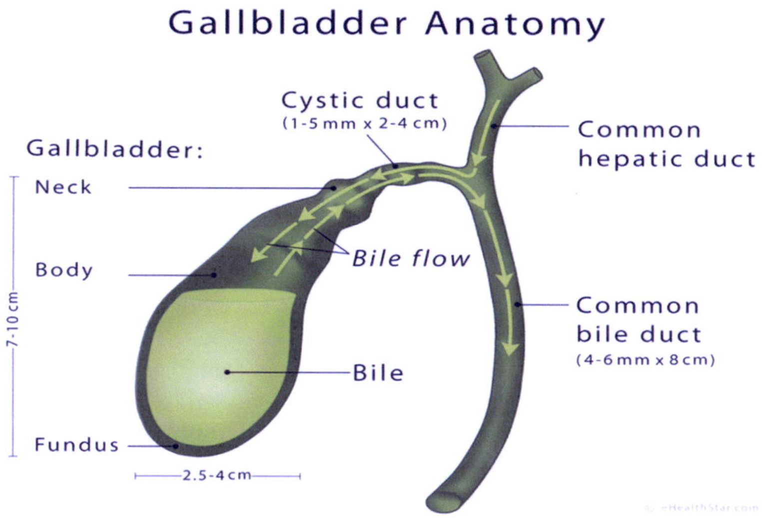

Figure 2.
Gallbladder parts and bile ducts (Jan Modric, 2017) [5].

As previously stated, the right posterior duct connects to the right anterior duct and unites it from the left to produce the right hepatic duct, which then connects to the left hepatic duct to form the common hepatic duct. The most prevalent anatomic variant of the biliary system is drainage of the right posterior duct into the left hepatic duct before its confluence with the right anterior duct.

Furthermore, various less common and usually more difficult anatomic variants of the bile ducts, which include both aberrant and auxiliary bile ducts, have been described. In a clinical setting, knowing the difference between an aberrant bile duct and an accessory bile duct is vital since an aberrant bile duct is the only bile duct draining a specific hepatic segment, whereas an accessory bile duct drains the same portion of the liver. Failure to recognize certain of these bile duct irregularities can lead to bile leakage and peritoneal membrane irritation (bile peritonitis). Endoscopic retrograde cholangiopancreatography is used to treat these leaks by inserting stents (ERCP). They can stop these leaks that arise from the common bile or cystic ducts [8–10].

4. The sphincter of Oddi: (anatomy and physiology)

The human sphincter of Oddi is approximately 10 mm in length and has a well-defined and strong musculature. The Oddi sphincter is physically and functionally distinct from the duodenum. Its myoelectrical and contractile patterns are distinct from those of the duodenum in terms of character and timing. The contractions of the human sphincter of Oddi occur at the same time; however, there may be minor variations in configuration that look peristaltic at times. Its principal function of serving as a bile flow resistor is compatible with the occurrence of synchronous contractions. Because of the sphincter of Oddi resistance, the constant hepatic production of bile is largely directed into the cystic duct and gallbladder during the fasting state, where it is stored and concentrated. During the diastolic phase, sphincter of Oddi phasic contractions and, during phase II, migrating motor complex occur when there is modest gallbladder contraction; hence, a tiny amount of bile escapes into the duodenum. The gallbladder contracts during digestion, emptying the majority of its contents, and bile is delivered to the duodenum *via* the cystic and common bile ducts, which pass *via* a relaxed sphincter of Oddi and duodenum. Bile salts help in fat digestion and absorption in the duodenum and jejunum (triglycerides, cholesterol and phospholipids, and liposoluble vitamins). Therefore, transportation of bile salts to the terminal ileum takes place; there, most of them were recycled as part of the enterohepatic circulation through an active transport mechanism found in the terminal ileum's epithelial cells [6].

5. Sphincter of Oddi dyskinesia

Patients with sphincter of Oddi (SO) dyskinesia have biliary-like symptoms, which are frequently noticed after a cholecystectomy. The symptoms and signs of bile duct sphincter dysfunction are similar to those of temporary bile duct blockage, whereas pancreatic sphincter of Oddi dysfunction is linked to elevated pancreatic enzymes and even full-blown pancreatitis. Patients with sphincter of Oddi dysfunction are assessed with quantitative choledochoscintigraphy and/or sphincter of Oddi manometry tests to confirm the diagnosis, even if the preliminary investigation is defined by this functional entity by sphincter of Oddi manometry.

6. Chronic and acute cholecystitis

6.1 Pathogenesis

The most commonly stated hypothesis in the etiology of chronic and acute cholecystitis is that it is caused by gallstones migrating from the gallbladder obstructing the cystic duct or, in the event of big gallstones, that they intermittently obstruct the gallbladder's neck (Jose Behar) [6]. The inability to see the gallbladder in patients with acute cholecystitis has been attributed to a cystic duct occlusion. This observation has been validated clinically and pathologically in up to 97% of individuals with acute cholecystitis [Pare and Shaffer et al.] [11].

However, other explanations for this failure are more likely that.

A cystic duct obstruction would be caused by the gallbladder's acute inflammation and edema spreading to the cystic duct, or.

Because it is clogged with inflammatory fluids, an atonic gallbladder obstructs the entry of the bulk of the isotope-labeled agent. Furthermore, the severely inflamed gallbladder may be unable to distend passively due to edema or actively due to a faulty relaxation found in gallbladders with lithogenic bile containing high cholesterol contents [Xiao and Chen et al.] [12].

The appearance of cholecystitis associated only with lithogenic bile (acalculous gallbladder) or a single huge stone several times larger than the normal width of the cystic duct lumen further challenges the idea of cystic duct obstruction. Furthermore, the presence of acute inflammation on top of a chronically inflamed or atrophic fibrotic gallbladder has proven difficult to explain because it would imply recurring cystic duct obstruction events. It is more likely that the development of acute inflammation as a result of a chronic process had been in the works for a long time. Mucosal thickening, hypertrophic muscle layers, and macrophage infiltration of the lamina propria are common in gallbladders. In the absence of gallstones, chronic cholecystitis is commonly found histopathologically. They arise in people who are morbidly obese and have lithogenic bile but no gallstones. When compared with the normal mucosa in nonobese people, these gallbladders exhibit mucosal abnormalities consistent with chronic cholecystitis [Csendes et al.] [13]. The pathogenesis of chronic cholecystitis is shown in **Figure 3**. The gallbladder

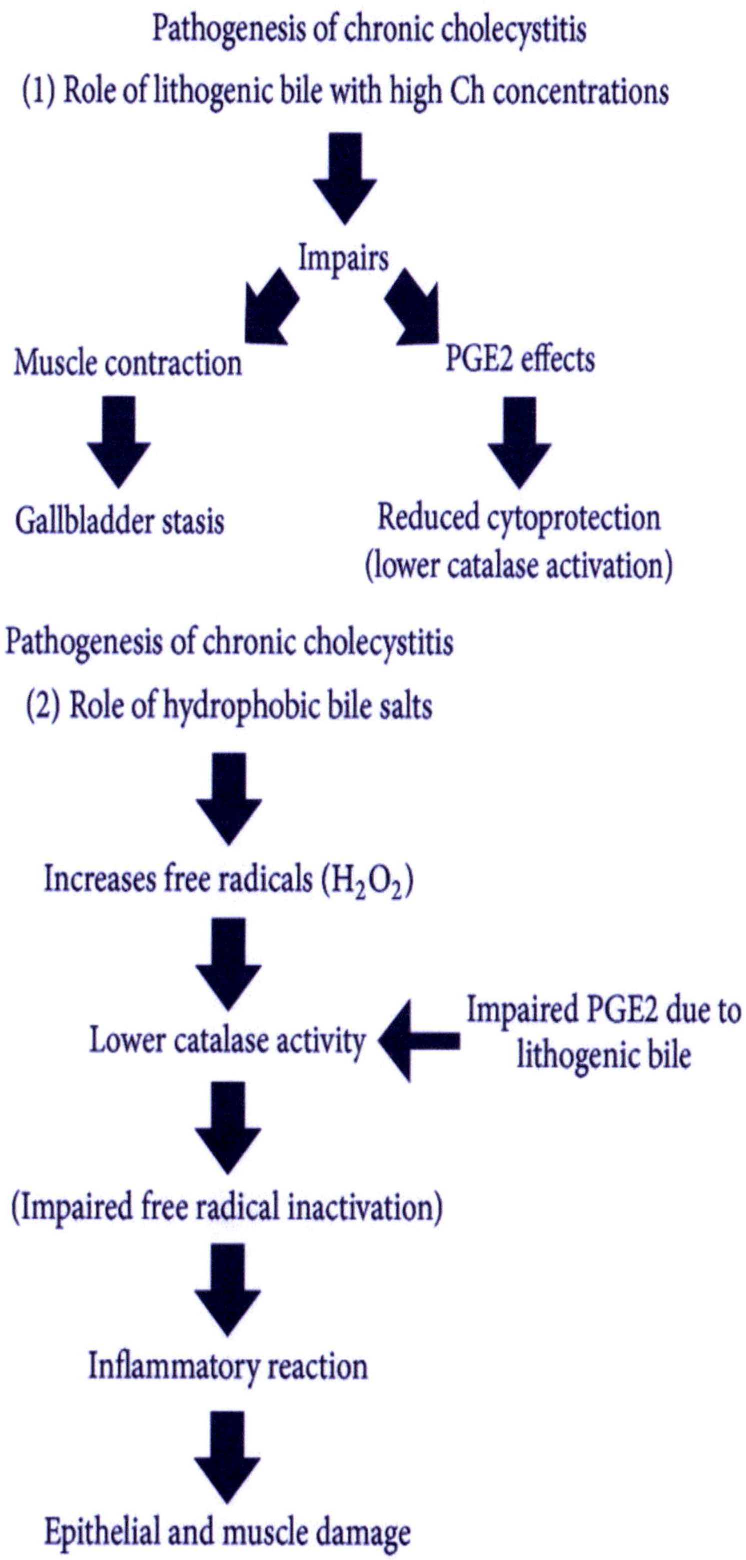

Figure 3.
Pathogenesis of chronic cholecystitis.

motility and cytoprotective functions are impaired by lithogenic hepatic bile with excess cholesterol, allowing the hydrophobic bile salts to induce chronic cholecystitis.

Finally, the results of the aforementioned human and animal studies strongly suggest that cholecystitis develops in the presence of lithogenic bile with high cholesterol concentrations, which creates a permissive environment for hydrophobic bile salts to increase oxidative stress levels and initiate the inflammatory process. Continuous entrance of hydrophobic bile salts into the diseased gallbladder is required for this inflammatory process [14].

7. Chronic cholecystitis clinical symptoms

Chronic cholecystitis patients may be asymptomatic or experience recurring episodes of epigastric and right upper quadrant (RUQ) discomfort that radiates often around the waist and toward the scapula. The pain is moderate to severe, and it is not postprandial but rather nocturnal in nature. It does not happen every day; instead, it happens every two to 3 weeks. Ultrasonography is usually used to make the diagnosis. Gallstones and gallbladder wall thickening can be detected using this test. Laboratory tests are normal. Gallstones are often asymptomatic, but because they are easily discovered in gallbladders by imaging investigations, they are blamed for a range of upper gastrointestinal problems. Gallstones are frequently blamed for nonspecific gastrointestinal symptoms such as persistent dyspepsia, gastroparesis, and irritable bowel syndrome. Patients with these functional disorders typically experience everyday upper gastrointestinal symptoms, which are often postprandial and triggered by fatty foods or large meals. Epigastric pain, nausea, and bloating are common complaints among these patients. Even while pathological investigations may indicate gallstones and histological evidence of persistent cholecystitis, cholecystectomy does not relieve these symptoms. Gallstones can go unnoticed for lengthy periods of time, according to several investigations, including autopsy studies. Most patients with asymptomatic gallstones remained symptom free for the whole 8-year follow-up period in a prospective Italian research [15–19].

8. Acute cholecystitis

In acute cholecystitis, chronic cholecystitis is the most prevalent risk factor. These patients often have abrupt onset of severe pain, which is commonly accompanied by nausea in 90% of instances and vomiting in 50% of cases.

Physical examination indicates epigastric, right upper quadrant, and positive Murphy sign pain, with rebound soreness in severe instances. However, doctors must rule out other acute abdominal diseases such as acute appendicitis, particularly with a retrocecal appendix, acute pancreatitis, localized perforated peptic ulcer, intestinal perforation, or ischemia before considering this diagnosis. These clinical entities exhibit comparable characteristics in terms of demographics and risk factors. Physical examination indicates abdominal pain that can be localized or widespread, as well as a significant decrease in bowel sounds, in these individuals who complain of severe stomach pain, nausea, and vomiting.

Acute cholecystitis is defined as an acute inflammation of the gall bladder. Chronic cholecystitis, acute pancreatitis, diverticulitis, colitis, appendicitis, Fitz-Hugh-Curtis syndrome, ureteral stone, and omental infarction are all illnesses that can cause acute right upper quadrant (RUQ) discomfort [20, 21]. It can occur abruptly in conjunction with gallstones (acute calculous cholecystitis) or less frequently without gallstones (acute calculous cholecystitis) (acalculous cholecystitis). Gallstones affect more than 80% of persons who are asymptomatic. Acute cholecystitis is a complication of gallstone disease that usually arises in people who have had symptomatic gallstones in the past. Delayed management can lead to increased morbidity, due to progression to severe cholecystitis, such as gangrenous change, abscess formation, and gallbladder perforation [4].

9. Microorganisms in biliary tract infections

The majority of cases of acute cholecystitis are caused by an impacted gallstone blocking the gallbladder outlet, resulting in an increase in intraluminal pressure, gallbladder distension, and wall edema, and eventually gallbladder necrosis. During the early stages of acute cholecystitis, bile is normally sterile, and infection occurs as a side effect.

Biliary tract infection is a prevalent cause of bacteremia and is linked to a high rate of morbidity and mortality, especially in elderly individuals with comorbid conditions or when diagnosis and treatment are delayed. Enterobacteriaceae, which climb from the gastrointestinal system, are the most prevalent infectious organisms. Complications such as acute renal failure and septic shock are more likely in patients with bacteremia.

9.1 Bacterial causes of biliary tract infections

The most frequently identified pathogens are Gram-negative microorganisms, primarily *Escherichia coli*, *Salmonella enteritidis*, *Acinetobacter baumannii*, *Citrobacter freundii*, *Enterobacter cloacae*, and *Klebsiella* species. Within Gram-positive microorganisms, *Clostridium perfringens* is most commonly observed. Previous research has linked biliary infection with gallstone development and indicated that bacteria may act as the nucleating factor initiating the formation of both pigment and cholesterol gallstones. Many studies [22, 23] had established the coexistence of biofilm-forming bacteria in bile and gallbladder/gallstones (*Pseudomonas aeruginosa, E. coli, Klebsiella pneumoniae, Enterococcus* spp. and *Acinetobacter* spp.) in different combinations, and the presence of *Capnocytophaga* spp., *Lactococcus* spp., *Bacillus* spp., *Staphylococcus haemolyticus*, *Enterobacter* or *Citrobacter* spp., *Morganella* spp., *Salmonella* spp., and *Helicobacter pylori*.

All of the microbiological studies that led to the selection of these antibiotic regimens were carried out using standard culture methods. Recent studies of microbial detection by culture- vs. culture-free identification of microbial DNA by next-generation sequencing (NGS) for various purulent diseases have shown that traditional culture only identifies a portion of the bacteria present. Additionally, in some Asian countries, the presence of *H. pylori* has been detected infrequently in the gallbladder by PCR. Other molecular tools like RAPD fingerprinting, *cagA* gene detection, which represent a good marker for genome-sequencing projects, are available nowadays to detect the microbial strains causing infections in AC patients [24].

9.2 ESKAPE pathogens and role of bile in development of drug resistance

Bile has bactericidal activity. However, many pathogens are known to resist the bactericidal activity of bile and utilize this host component as a localization signal to regulate virulence gene expression and enhance infection. Furthermore, strategies employed by pathogens to resist bile align with antibiotic resistance mechanisms. The efflux pump genes, *acrAB* in *E. coli*, *Salmonella*, *Shigella*, *Klebsiella*, and other pathogens, resist both bile salts and antibiotics, thereby making it essential for survival under extreme environmental conditions [25–28].

The ESKAPE group of pathogens (*Enterococcus, Staphylococcus, Klebsiella, Acinetobacter, Pseudomonas, and* Enterobacter) represents a significant public health threat as antibiotic resistance rates rise from the acquisition of multiple resistance mechanisms involving the gene expression of BSH, Gls24, GlsB, EmrB/QacA, PrkC, LiaFSR, BsrXRS, MnhF, WTA, OxyR, CpxAR, KpnO, KpnEF, CadC, TdcA, Gal ET, *pgaABCD*, *pqsABCDE*, ExoU, T6SS genes or through biofilm production, etc. Many ESKAPE pathogens are not known to cause infection in the gastrointestinal system; nevertheless, isolation from bile, the gallbladder, pancreatic or biliary stent biofilms, and bile duct infections have been described, and antibiotic resistance is frequently identified. Given a previous research that found positive bile cultures in 22.2% of the cases following elective gallbladder removal surgery, the findings are not restricted to hospital-based infections. Enterococcus spp. was the most frequent bacterial isolate found in the bile samples, followed by *E. coli*, *Klebsiella* spp., *Enterobacter* spp., and *Pseudomonas* spp.; 22.7% of these isolates were antibiotic-resistant. Furthermore, bile exposure in the lungs of CF patients has been shown to affect *Staphylococcus aureus, A. baumannii,* and especially *P. aeruginosa* infection. Growth was either consistent or increased in the presence of human bile, respectively, for *E. coli* or *Enterococcus faecalis*. Furthermore, bile reduced the antimicrobial activity of ciprofloxacin, meropenem, and tigecycline for *E. coli*, while linezolid and tigecycline had reduced activity against *E. faecalis* [29].

9.3 Rare cases of acute cholecystitis caused by microorganisms

Berinson et al. [30] reported one rare case of AC caused by *Kosakonia cowanii*, formerly known as *Enterobacter cowanii*, which is a Gram-negative bacillus belonging to the order *Enterobacterales*. The species is usually recognized as a plant pathogen and has only anecdotally been encountered as a human pathogen. A cholecystectomy confirmed the diagnosis of acute cholecystitis with partial gall bladder necrosis. By MALDI-TOF, 16S-rRNA analysis, and whole-genome sequencing, a surgical material produced pure cultures of Gram-negative rods that were clearly identified as K. cowanii.

Deering et al. [31] reported a rare case of acute cholecystitis caused by *Streptococcus bovis* biotypes (I & II), a Gram-positive, catalase-negative, anaerobic coccus found as a commensal inhabitant of the digestive system in 16% of healthy people. The patient was treated with tazobactam/piperacillin and later on subjected to laparoscopic cholecystectomy.

Vogt et al. [32] reported isolated Serogroup O1 *Vibrio cholerae* in an 83-year-old man suffering from AC. The Gram stain of the body fluid specimen demonstrated rare Gram-negative rods and many polymorphonuclear lymphocytes. The organism was positive for oxidase, and the results obtained using a Neg Breakpoint Combo Panel Type 41 (NBC41) and a MicroScan WalkAway Plus system (Siemens Healthcare Diagnostics, Deerfield, IL) identified the organism as *V. cholerae*, with 97.76% probability. The isolate was also tested using a manual API 20E Gram-negative identification panel (bioMerieux, Inc.,), which yielded a code of 5,347,124, giving a presumptive identification of *V. cholerae* at 99.9%.

9.4 Viral causes of biliary tract infections

In comparison with bacterial infections, viral infections of the biliary tract are less common and less discussed. Viral infections frequently occur as a result of a liver infection or as part of a systemic viral illness. Viruses seldom cause primary liver infection. Cholangitis, or inflammation of the bile duct, is a very frequent symptom. Despite the fact that hepatotropic viruses (A, B, C, and E) are commonly thought of as hepatocellular pathogens, cholangitic symptoms are now widely documented in conjunction with these disorders [10, 14, 23, 33]. Cholangitis is also due to systemic viral infections in different proportions to hepatitis. The human immunodeficiency virus (HIV) is linked to a variety of liver problems, including cholangitis. Other systemic viruses, most notably members of the herpes virus family, can induce hepatic illness in both immunocompromised and immunocompetent individuals, including cholangitis and potentially ductopenia [34].

9.5 Parasitic causes of biliary tract infections

Cholangitis can be caused due to a variety of reasons, including biliary calculi, strictures, parasites, post-endoscopic retrograde cholangiopancreatography (ERCP), postoperative, and so on. Biliary parasitoses, in contrast to other causes, are more prevalent in many nations. Ascaris lumbricoides, liver flukes, and Echinococcus are common parasites that affect the biliary system. The trematodes (flukes) that commonly infect the human biliary tract include *Clonorchis sinensis, Opisthorchis viverrini, Opisthorchis felineus, and Fasciola hepatica.* The majority of patients are asymptomatic. While entering through the bile duct, they cause biliary colic and obstructive jaundice. The parasites reside in the intrahepatic bile ducts and, occasionally, in the extrahepatic bile ducts, gallbladder, and pancreatic duct. The result is mechanical obstruction, inflammatory reaction, adenomatous hyperplasia, and periductal fibrosis. The parasite can be examined through radiological findings of CT and MRI [35].

9.6 Diagnosis

The diagnostic criteria include examining for signs of local inflammation, such as Murphy's sign, the presence of a mass, pain, or tenderness located in the upper right quadrant of the abdomen. The local inflammation is often accompanied by systemic inflammation, indicated by signs of fever, increased white blood cell (WBC) counts, and elevated levels of C-reactive protein. The severity of acute cholecystitis can range from mild and self-limiting to severe and potentially life threatening [36, 37]. Several imaging techniques such as ultrasonography, magnetic resonance imaging (MRI), computed tomography (CT) are necessary to accurately diagnose both the typical and atypical cases of acute cholecystitis. Recently, Amini et al. had used high mobility group box protein 1 (HMGB1) biomarker for acute cholecystitis diagnosis [38].

9.6.1 Diagnosis of cholecystitis

For the consensus in diagnosis of cholecystitis in 2007, the Tokyo guidelines for the management of acute cholangitis and cholecystitis (TG07) were formed and widely adopted. In 2013, the updated Tokyo guidelines (TG13) for acute cholangitis and acute cholecystitis were released for severity grading of acute cholecystitis [37] (**Table 1**).

9.6.2 TG07 severity assessment criteria

The severity assessment criteria were first presented throughout the world in TG07 by Hirota and Takada, [37] where the severity grading of acute cholecystitis

Local signs of inflammation, etc. Murphy's sign RUQ Mass/pain/tenderness
Systemic signs of inflammation, etc. Fever Elevated CRP Elevated WBC count
Imaging findings Imaging findings characteristic of acute cholecystitis
Suspected diagnosis: One item in A + one item in B Definitive diagnosis: One item in A + one item in B + C
Acute hepatitis, other acute abdominal diseases, and chronic cholecystitis should be excluded. RUQ-right upper abdominal quadrant, CRP-C-reactive protein, WBC-white blood cell.

Table 1.
TG13 diagnostic criteria for acute cholecystitis.

was classified into the following three categories: "mild (Grade I)," "moderate (Grade II)," and "severe (Grade III)."

Mild (Grade I) acute cholecystitis occurred in a patient with no signs of organ failure and mild gallbladder illness, allowing cholecystectomy to be performed safely and with minimal risk. The severity score for these individuals in TG07 does not fulfill the criteria for "moderate (Grade II)" and "severe (Grade III)" acute cholecystitis.

Acute cholecystitis, in which the degree of acute inflammation is expected to be linked with greater operating difficulties in completing cholecystectomy, was classified as moderate (Grade II) acute cholecystitis [8, 9, 16].

Severe (Grade III) acute cholecystitis was defined as acute cholecystitis associated with organ dysfunction (**Table 2**).

Reference: Masamichi et al. [19].

9.7 Treatment

Acute cholecystitis is often treated promptly by cholecystectomy or percutaneous cholecystostomy and antibiotic therapy in high-risk patients. Antimicrobial treatment has a different role depending on the severity of the illness and its etiology. Because it is unclear if bacteria have a role in grade I acute cholecystitis, antimicrobial treatment is used to prevent infection before cholecystectomy. Antimicrobial treatment is therapeutic and necessary for grade II acute cholecystitis until the gallbladder is removed. Most patients with bacteremia might have clinical deterioration and can be classified as grade III acute cholecystitis and are therefore not suitable for surgery. A recent meta-analysis reported that cholecystography has the highest diagnostic accuracy for detection of acute cholecystitis [39].

Previous studies have found bile to be infected in 9–42% of patients who underwent elective laparoscopic cholecystectomy, but the incidence of culture-positive bile increased to 35–65% of patients with acute cholecystitis [40]. Antimicrobial treatment is critical for reducing both the systemic septic response and local inflammation following cholecystectomy in individuals with moderate-to-severe acute cholecystitis [41]. Those with septic shock should get appropriate antibiotic treatment within 1 hour of diagnosis, and patients who are less severely sick should receive it within 6 hours. Bile culture results, however, cannot be acquired promptly after admission, and bile culture necessitates percutaneous gallbladder puncture. As a result, the most successful empiric antibiotics described in the literature are used as the basis for first antimicrobial treatment [42].

Associated with dysfunction of any one of the following organ/systems	
Cardiovascular dysfunction	**Hypotension requiring treatment with dopamine >5 ub/kg per min, or any dose of norepinephrine**
Neurologic dysfunction	Decreased level of consciousness
Respiratory dysfunction	Pa2O/FiO2 ratio < 300
Renal dysfunction	Oluguria, creatinine >2.0 mg/dl
Hepatic dysfunction	PT – INR > 1.5
Hematological dysfunction	Platelet count <100,000/mm^3
Grade II (moderate) acute cholecystitis	
Associated with any one of the following conditions: 1. Elevated white blood cell count ([18,000/mm^3) 2. Palpable tender mass in the right upper abdominal quadrant 3. Duration of complaints (72 h) 4. Marked local inflammation (gangrenous cholecystitis, pericholecystic abscess, hepatic abscess, biliary peritonitis, and emphysematous cholecystitis)	
Grade I (mild) acute cholecystitis	
Does not meet the criteria of "Grade III" or "Grade II" acute cholecystitis. Grade I can also be defined as acute cholecystitis in a healthy patient with no organ dysfunction and mild inflammatory changes in the gallbladder, making cholecystectomy a safe and low-risk operative procedure.	

Table 2.
TG 13 severity grading for acute cholecystitis.

Because most infections in acute cholecystitis are limited to the gallbladder, sampling should be done directly from the infection site in order to identify the true causative pathogen. Bile specimens collected from the biliary tract using percutaneous transhepatic biliary drainage (PTBD) or endoscopic nasobiliary drainage (ENBD) are potentially associated with microbial contamination [43].

Bacterial infection is commonly reported in 50 to 90% of the cases. Most of the studies reported the involvement of polymicrobial infections in AC, which were often treated with antibiotic regimens with two or more antibiotics, but only one study had reported that monomicrobial growth was involved in AC. The most common presumptive antibiotics used in AC are ceftriaxone (2gm, IV, OD) or piperacillin/tazobactam (4.5 gm, IV, 8 hourly) or cefoperazone/sulbactam (3gm, IV, 12 hourly) for 7 to 10 days. The second-line or alternative antibiotics is imipenem (500 mg, IV, 6 hourly) or meropenem (1gm, IV, 8hourly) for 7 to 10 days. The most commonly isolated microorganisms among pathogens in positive bile cultures are Enterococci species, non-*faecium* enterococci (*Enterococcus faecalis*, *Enterococcus gallinarum*, *Enterococcus casseliflavus*, *Enterococcus avium*), *Escherichia Coli*, and *Klebsiella* species [44]. Gram-positive microbes, such as Enterococci, have become less common over time, whereas Gram-negative germs, particularly Enterobacteriales, have become more common and are most typically isolated among patients with acute cholecystitis. The results of local antimicrobial susceptibility tests, as well as information of the likely infecting microorganisms, pharmacokinetics/pharmacodynamics, and adverse reactions/effects of available medicines, must all be considered when making antimicrobial therapy decisions (local antibiogram). The severity of the illness and previous antimicrobial exposure are also important considerations in deciding the best course of treatment. β-lactam antibiotics or their derivatives, cephalosporins, carbapenems, fluoroquinolones, and other antibiotics diminish infection. For moderate and severe acute cholecystitis, empiric treatment with piperacillin/tazobactam or a cephalosporin with or without metronidazole is advised, regardless of whether or not there is growth on culture [45].

Broad-spectrum β-lactam and β-lactamase inhibitors, such as ampicillin-sulbactam, have been recommended as the first-line drugs to treat Enterococci and non-*faecium* enterococci infections. However, these microorganisms are reported to be resistant to most of the classes of antibiotics represented earlier. VREFM (vancomycin-resistant *Enterococcus faecium*) was reported for the first time in 2021 by Suk-Won et al. [46]. The authors found that the majority of the patients were suffering from Grade II acute cholecystitis (94.7%). Hence, they recommended other antibiotics, such as linezolid and tigecycline, which provide good coverage against VREFM, should be considered for patients with such advanced infections. Tigecycline can be used in several other cases because of its broad spectrum of effectiveness against Gram-negative microorganisms, including ESBL-producing bacteria. Tasina et al. [47] reported poor effectiveness of tigecycline toward a severely ill patient with AC.

Piperacillin-tazobactam and third- or fourth-generation cephalosporins are indicated as first-line antibiotics for Gram-negative bacteria, with fluoroquinolones and carbapenems as second-line antibiotics, depending on the severity of the infection and antimicrobial susceptibility patterns. According to Gomi et al. [48], most identified strains were resistant to ciprofloxacin due to widespread use of the antibiotic by the community, whereas 20% of pathogenic bacteria were resistant to ceftriaxone. As a result, in such circumstances, piperacillin-tazobactam or cefepime, which have larger spectra and lower resistance rates, are indicated. Carbapenem and tigecycline are advised for patients who are taking antibiotics on a regular basis. However, because of widespread medication resistance and associated high morbidity and mortality rates, carbapenem-resistant strains (CRE) species have emerged as major healthcare-related diseases [49].

9.7.1 Empiric antibiotic treatment of community-acquired biliary tract infections (CA-BTI)

The most important approach in controlling the CA-BTI is the primary source controls such as biliary drainage, removal of biliary tract stones, and cholecystectomy. The primary source control can help the antibiotics to penetrate the biliary tract, resulting in a better bactericidal effect when biliary obstruction is present. While it comes to medical therapy, there are two crucial variables to consider when choosing empiric antibiotics. Administration of antibiotics is essential for the treatment of BTI, in addition to primary source control. As the BTI is caused by endogenous etiological agents, that is, gastrointestinal tract flora, such as Escherichia coli, Klebsiella spp., Enterococci spp., Bacteroides spp., antibiotics that are effective against these organisms are usually used empirically to treat BTI rather than definite therapy. However, the usage of inappropriate empiric antibiotics may also incur fatal outcomes. To elicit positive treatment responses, >80% of the presumed causative microorganisms should be sensitive to antibiotics, and for patients with septic shock, the susceptibility rates should even exceed 100% [50]. Next, the antibiotics must be present in adequate concentrations at the infection sites to have the desired antimicrobial action [51, 52]. **Table 3** shows the antibiotics usually used to treat biliary tract infections based on their biliary penetration ability (indicated by the ratio of bile-to-serum concentrations [53–55].

Augmentin = amoxicillin + clavulanate; Bile/serum = bile concentration/serum concentration; Tazocin: Piperacillin + tazobactum; Unasyn = ampicillin + sulbactum.

Good penetration efficiency (>1)		**Low-penetration efficiency (<1)**	
Antibiotics	**Bile/serum**	**Antibiotics**	**Bile/serum**
Tazocin	60	Cefotaxime	0.75
Tigecycline	38	Meropenem	0.75
Augmentin	30	Ceftazidime	0.5
Ciprofloxacin	30	Vancomycin	0.5
Unasyn	9	Amikacin	0.3
Ceftriaxone	5	Gentamycin	0.3
Levofloxacin	5	Cefipime	0.1
Penicillin G	5	Imepenem	0.01
Cefazolin	3		
Clindamycin	3		
Doripenem	1.17		
Cefuroxime	1		
Metronidazole	1		

Table 3.
Antibiotics frequently used to treat biliary tract infections and their biliary penetration ability (indicated as the ration of bile to serum concentrations).

As a result, when choosing empiric antibiotics for the treatment of BTI, both susceptibility rates and the potential of biliary penetration should be taken into account. **Table 3** lists the antibiotics often used to treat BTI, as well as their biliary penetration ability (measured as the ratio of bile-to-serum concentrations). Only individuals with a reasonable ratio (>1) of bile-to-serum concentrations (**Table 3**) could be candidates for empiric antibiotics for BTI, according to the criteria outlined earlier. The local antimicrobial susceptibility patterns of the usual causative agents for BTI should also be considered when prescribing appropriate empiric antibiotics. To ensure a positive outcome, only those with a 20% resistance rate should be used as empirical antibiotics.

Patients with severe cholecystitis are unfortunately difficult to identify effectively, both clinically and radiologically, because clinical presentations are unpredictable, and imaging findings are frequently ambiguous. However, there are significant differences in morbidity and fatality rates between patients with uncomplicated cholecystitis and those with severe cholecystitis. Preventing related consequences requires early detection and careful management of patients at risk of severe cholecystitis.

10. Conclusions

When acute cholecystitis is suspected, bile samples are taken for microbiology culture and sensitivity testing, and antibiotics are prescribed once the diagnosis has been established. The antibiotics of choice are parenteral cephalosporin or ampicillin, as well as aminoglycosides. The antibiotic regimen chosen is based on the severity of the clinical presentation. Because acute suppurative cholangitis with biliary blockage has a high pre- and postoperative mortality rate, comprehensive antimicrobial therapy is required following biliary decompression. Bile microbiological analysis is an expedient diagnostic tool for determining more suitable medication and generating local antibiotic guidelines for the treatment of biliary tract infections.

Conflict of interest

No potential conflict of interest was reported by the authors.

Author details

Hema Prakash Kumari Pilli* and Vijayalakshmi Payala
Department of Clinical Microbiology, GITAM Institute of Medical Sciences and Research, GITAM deemed to be University, Rushikonda, Visakhapatnam, India

*Address all correspondence to: hemaprakashpilli@gmail.com

References

[1] Everhart JE, Khare M, Hill M, et al. Prevalence and ethnic differences in gallstone disease in the United States. Gastroenteriology. 1999;**117**:632-639

[2] Sifri CD, Madoff LC. Infections of the liver and biliary system. In: Mandell GI, Je B, Dolin R, editors. Mandell, Douglas and Bennett's Principles and Practice of Infectious Diseases. 7th ed. Churchill Livingstone Elsevier; 2010

[3] Indar AA, Beckingham JJ. Acute cholecystitis. BMJ. 2002;**325**:639-643

[4] Wadhwa V, Jobanputra Y, Garg SK, Patwardhan S, Mehta D, Sanaka MR. Nationwide trends of hospital admissions for acute cholecystitis in the United States. Gastroenterology Report (Oxf). 2017;**5**(1):36-42. DOI: 10.1093/gastro/gow015

[5] Jan Modric. Gallbladder Anatomy and Function. 2017. Available from: https://www.google.com/url?sa=i&url=https%3A%2F%2Fwww.ehealthstar.com%2Fanatomy%2Fgallbladder&psig=AOvVaw0Bbqz_bOLIoCUjv1R7KeBM&ust=1625739131352000&source=images&cd=vfe&ved=2ahUKEwi4rNKs3NDxAhUHGCsKHfKRCRkQr4kDegQIARBc

[6] Behar J. Physiology and pathophysiology of the biliary tract: The gallbladder and sphincter of Oddi-a review. ISRN Physiology. 2013;**2013**:1-15. DOI: 10.1155/2013/837630

[7] Mortele KJ, Ros PR. Anatomic variants of the biliary tree: MR cholangiographic findings and clinical applications. American Journal of Roentgenology. 2001;**177**(2):389-394

[8] Brodsky A, Matter I, Sabo E, Cohen A, Abrahamson J, Eldar S. Laparoscopic cholecystectomy for acute cholecystitis: Can the need for conversion and the probability of complications be predicted? A prospective study. Surgical Endoscopy. 2000;**14**:755-60. 45

[9] Teixeira JP, Sraiva AC, Cabral AC, Barros H, Reis JR, Teixeira A. Conversion factors in laparoscopic cholecystectomy for acute cholecystitis. Hepato-Gastroenterology. 2000;**47**:626-30. 46

[10] Rosh A, Manko J. Cholangitis. Available from: eMedicine.com. 2006

[11] Pare P, Shaffer EA, Rosenthall L. Nonvisualization of the gallbladder by 99m Tc-HIDA cholescintigraphy as evidence of cholecystitis. Canadian Medical Association Journal. 1978;**118**(4):384-386

[12] Xiao ZL, Chen Q, Amaral J, Biancani P, Behar J. Defect of receptor-G protein coupling in human gallbladder with cholesterol stones. American Journal of Physiology. 2000;**278**(2):G251-G258

[13] Csendes A, Burdiles P, Smok G, Csendes P, Burgos A, Recio M. Histologic findings of gallbladder mucosa in 87 patients with morbid obesity without gallstones compared to 87 control subjects. Journal of Gastrointestinal Surgery. 2003;**4**(7):547-551

[14] Kinney TP. Management of ascending cholangitis. Gastrointestinal Endoscopy Clinics of North America. 2007;**17**:289-306

[15] Jones MW, Gnanapandithan K, Panneerselvam D, et al. Chronic Cholecystitis. Treasure Island (FL): StatPearls Publishing; 2021

[16] Rattner DW, Ferguson C, Warshaw AL. Factors associated with successful laparoscopic cholecystectomy for acute cholecystitis. Annals of Surgery. 1993;**217**:233-6. 48

[17] Araujo-Teixeria JP, Rocha-Reis J, Costa-Cabral A, Barros H, Saraiva AC, Araujo-Teixeira AM. Laparoscopic versus open cholecystectomy for cholecystitis (200 cases). Comparison of results and predictive factors for conversion. Chirurgie. 1999;**124**:529-535 (in French with English abstract). 49.

[18] Merriam LT, Kanaan SA, Dawes JG, Angelos P, Prystowsky JB, Rege RV, et al. Gangrenous cholecystitis: Analysis of risk factors and experience with laparoscopic cholecystectomy. Surgery. 1999;**126**:680-685

[19] Masamichi Y, Tadahiro T, Steven MS, et al. TG13 diagnostic criteria and severity grading of acute cholecystitis (with videos). Journal of Hepato-Biliary-Pancreatic Sciences. 2013;**20**:35-46

[20] Hanbidge AE, Buckler PM, O'Malley ME, et al. From the RSNA refresher courses: Imaging evaluation for acute pain in the right upper quadrant. Radiographics. 2004;**24**: 1117-1135

[21] Kim SW, Kim HC, Yang DM, et al. Cystic duct enhancement: a useful CT finding in the diagnosis of acute cholecystitis without visible impacted gallstones. AJR. American Journal of Roentgenology. 2015;**205**:991-998

[22] Lee CC, Chang IJ, Lai YC, et al. Epidemiology and prognostic determinants of patients with bacteraemic cholecystitis or cholangitis. The American Journal of Gastroenterology. 2007;**102**:563-569

[23] Flores C, Maguilnik I, Hadlich E, Goldani LZ. Microbiology of choledochal bile in patients with choledocholithiasis admitted to a tertiary hospital. Journal of Gastroenterology and Hepatology. 2003;**18**:333-336

[24] Backert S, Tegtmeyer N, Oyarzabal OA, et al. Unusual Manifestation of Live *Staphylococcus saprophyticus, Corynebacterium urinapleomorphum*, and *Helicobacter pylori* in the Gallbladder with Cholecystitis. International Journal of Molecular Sciences. 2018;**19**(7):1826. DOI: 10.3390/ijms19071826

[25] Pos KM. Drug transport mechanism of the AcrB efflux pump. Biochimica et Biophysica Acta. 2009;**1794**:782-793. DOI: 10.1016/j.bbapap.2008.12.015

[26] Seeger MA, Diederichs K, Eicher T, Brandstatter L, Schiefner A, Verrey F, et al. The AcrB efflux pump: conformational cycling and peristalsis lead to multidrug resistance. Current Drug Targets. 2008;**9**:729-749. DOI: 10.2174/138945008785747789

[27] Sistrunk JR, Nickerson KP, Chanin RB, Rasko DA, Faherty CS. Survival of the fittest: How bacterial pathogens utilize bile to enhance infection. Clinical Microbiology Reviews. 2016;**29**:819-836. DOI: 10.1128/CMR.00031-16

[28] Begley M, Gahan CG, Hill C. The interaction between bacteria and bile. FEMS Microbiology Reviews. 2005;**29**:625-651. DOI: 10.1016/j.femsre.2004.09.003

[29] Kevin Gipson S et al. The Great ESKAPE: Exploring the crossroads of bile and antibiotic resistance in bacterial pathogens. Infection and Immunity. 2020;**88**(10):5-19

[30] Berinson B, Bellon E, Christner M, Both A, Aepfelbacher M, Rohde H. Identification of Kosakonia cowanii as a rare cause of acute cholecystitis: Case report and review of the literature. BMC Infectious Diseases. 2020;**20**(1):366. DOI: 10.1186/s12879-020-05084-6

[31] Deering EM, Muravec Z, Castineira CF, O'Donoghue G. Streptococcus bovis-related cholecystitis. BML Case Reports.

2013;**2013**:bcr2013008581. DOI: 10.1136/bcr-2013-008581

[32] Vogt AP, Doshi RK, Higgins JE, Burd EM, Ribner BS, Kraft CS. Acute cholecystitis caused by nontoxigenic Vibrio cholerae O1 Inaba. Journal of Clinical Microbiology. 2010;**48**(3):1002-1004. DOI: 10.1128/JCM.02198-09

[33] Shivaprakasha S, Harish R, Dinesh KR, Karim PM. Aerobic bacterial isolates from choledochal bile at a tertiary hospital. Indian Journal of Pathology & Microbiology. 2006;**49**:464-467

[34] Gupta E, Anita C. Viral infections of the biliary tract. Saudi Journal of Gastroenterology. 2008;**14**(3):158-160

[35] Lim JH, Kim SY, Park CM. Parasitic diseases of the biliary tract. AJR. 2007;**188**:1596-1603

[36] Porter NL. Diseases of the gallbladder and bile ducts. Essentials. 2009;**64**

[37] Hirota M, Takada T, Kawarada Y, Nimura Y, Miura F, Hirata K, et al. Diagnostic criteria and severity assessment of acute cholecystitis: Tokyo guidelines. Journal of Hepato-Biliary-Pancreatic Surgery. 2007;**14**(1):78-82

[38] Amini M, Pakdaman A, Shapoori S, Mosayebi G. High mobility group box-1 (HMGB1) protein as a biomarker for acute cholecystitis. Reports of Biochemistry and Molecular Biology. 2019;**7**(2):204-209

[39] Pisano M et al. 2020 World Society of Emergency Surgery updated guidelines for the diagnosis and treatment of acute calculus cholecystitis. World Journal of Emergency Surgery. 2020;**15**:161. DOI: 10.1186/s13017-020-00336-x

[40] Ruan H-Q, Liao G-L, Peng P, Liu S-Q, et al. Microbial profiles and risk factors of preexisting biliary infection in patients with therapeutic endoscopy. Gastroenterology Research and Practice. 2019;**2019**:1527328, 8 pages. DOI: 10.1155/2019/1527328

[41] Rello J et al. Critical Care Infectious Diseases Textbook. Kluwer Academic Publishers; 2001

[42] Galili O et al. The effect of bactibilia on the course and outcome of laparoscopic cholecystectomy. European Journal of Clinical Microbiology & Infectious Diseases. 2008;**27**:797-803. DOI: 10.1007/s10096-008-0504-8

[43] Van den Hazel SJ, Speelman P, Tytgat GN, Dankert J, van Leeuwen DJ. Role of antibiotics in the treatment and prevention of acute and recurrent cholangitis. Clinical Infectious Diseases. 1994;**19**:279-286. DOI: 10.1093/clinids/19.2.279

[44] Rhodes A et al. Surviving sepsis campaign: International guidelines for management of sepsis and septic shock: 2016. Intensive Care Medicine. 2017;**43**:304-377. DOI: 10.1007/s00134-017-4683-6

[45] Yun SP, Seo HI. Clinical aspects of bile culture in patients undergoing laparoscopic cholecystectomy. Medicine. 2018;**97**:e11234. DOI: 10.1097/MD.0000000000011234

[46] Suh SW, Choi YS, Choi SH, et al. Antibiotic selection based on microbiology and resistance profiles of bile from gallbladder of patients with acute cholecystitis. Scientific Reports. 2021;**11**(1):2969. DOI: 10.1038/s41598-021-82603-8

[47] Tasina E, Haidich AB, Kokkali S, Arvanitidou M. Efficacy and safety of tigecycline for the treatment of infectious diseases: A meta-analysis. The Lancet Infectious Diseases. 2011;**11**:834-844. DOI: 10.1016/S1473-3099(11)70177-3

[48] Gomi H et al. Tokyo Guidelines 2018: Antimicrobial therapy for acute

cholangitis and cholecystitis. Journal of Hepato-Biliary-Pancreatic Sciences. 2018;**25**:3-16. DOI: 10.1002/jhbp.518

[49] Tischendorf J, de Avila RA, Safdar N. Risk of infection following colonization with carbapenem-resistant Enterobactericeae: A systematic review. American Journal of Infection Control. 2016;**44**:539-543. DOI: 10.1016/j.ajic.2015.12.005

[50] Bradley JS, Dudley MN, Drusano GL. Predicting efficacy of antiinfectives with pharmacodynamics and Monte Carlo simulation. The Pediatric Infectious Disease Journal. 2003;**22**:982e92

[51] Varghese JM, Roberts JA, Lipman J. Antimicrobial pharmacokinetic and pharmacodynamic issues in the critically ill with severe sepsis and septic shock. Critical Care Clinics. 2011;**27**:19e34

[52] Sharma S, Kumar A. Antimicrobial management of sepsis and septic shock. Clinics in Chest Medicine. 2008;**29**:677e87

[53] Cunha BA. Antibiotics essentials. In: Brogard JM, Pinget M, Arnaud JP, Dorner M, Lavillaureix J, editors. Biliary excretion of cefuroxime. Experimental and human study. Chemotherapy. 11th ed. Vol. 27. Burlington: Jones & Bartlett Learning; 2012, 1981. p. 526e718, 18e28

[54] Hukagawa H, Noga K. A study on the concentrations of levofloxacin in the gallbladder tissue and bile of patients. The Japanese Journal of Antibiotics. 1992;**45**:253e7

[55] Nielsen ML, Justesen T. Excretion of metroindazole in human bile. Investigations of hepatic bile, common duct bile, and gallbladder bile. Scandinavian Journal of Gastroenterology. 1977;**12**:1003-1008

Chapter 5

The Role of Endoscopic Ultrasound in Acute Cholecystitis

Cosmas Rinaldi A. Lesmana and Laurentius A. Lesmana

Abstract

Acute cholecystitis (AC) is one of challenging clinical conditions in biliary disorders as it can carry high morbidity and mortality. Gallstone disease is still the main cause of AC in clinical practice. Transabdominal ultrasound, abdominal CT scan and abdominal MRI are the standard diagnostic tools in AC, however, some obstacles can be found which are associated to the patient's factor, anatomy or anomaly of biliary system, the disease severity, and the operator. Cholecystectomy is still the primary choice management in AC condition, however, several issues need to be encountered, such as critically ill condition, sepsis, and patient's comorbidity. Percutaneous approach has become an alternative as it is considered as a simple procedure to be performed in clinical practice. Catheter dislodgement, the risk of bile leakage, and uncooperative patients have raised major concerns for this procedure. Another method, such as endoscopic approach has been studied as well and it seemed to have more advantage when compared to the percutaneous approach. Recently, endoscopic ultrasound (EUS) has been used as a combined diagnostic as well as therapeutic tools in managing biliary disorders. Recent evidences about the role of EUS approach for gallbladder drainage (EUS GBD) in patients who unsuitable for surgery have emerged in the past one decade. However, comprehensive evaluation before which approach is the best option is needed as expertise, cost, and patient's outcome prediction are the most important factors to be considered in the real clinical practice.

Keywords: acute cholecystitis, gallstone disease, surgical cholecystectomy, endoscopic ultrasound, gallbladder drainage

1. Introduction

Acute cholecystitis (AC) is one of challenging clinical condition due to acute inflammation of the gall bladder, where it can lead to severe and life-threatening condition. Gallstone disease is still the primary cause for AC, where it is estimated around 10–15% prevalence. Cholecystectomy is considered as the main choice of management in AC. However, there are many factors which involved in the management decision in clinical practice, such as early and late diagnosis of AC condition, whether it is mild, moderate, or severe, stone's location associated with the severity of inflammation and pain, bile duct inflammation (cholangitis), acute biliary pancreatitis, patient's comorbidity, and sepsis condition [1, 2]. Early diagnosis of acute cholecystitis is very important; however, it is not always possible as sometimes there is an incorrect time recognition by the patient or the family, the doctor's experience with the patient's symptoms, the quality of simple diagnostic tool (trans-abdominal ultrasound), and the ultrasound image's expertise [3, 4].

2. Acute cholecystitis diagnosis and the role of endoscopic ultrasound

Three modalities have been used in common clinical practice in diagnosing AC, which are transabdominal ultrasound (US), abdominal computed tomography (CT) scan, and abdominal magnetic resonance imaging (MRI) with cholangio-pancreatography (MRCP) [5]. Transabdominal US is considered as the easiest and fastest diagnostic tool to be performed bedside with very high sensitivity for gallbladder (GB) stone (cholelithiasis) detection, where gallstones can be identified more than 90% in AC. With this examination, it is very easy also to diagnose AC, confirmed by the abdominal-ultrasound pressure pain and thickening ("double layer") of the GB wall. However, this procedure has several limitations, such as obese patients, tiny stones detection, cystic duct evaluation, and it is still an operator dependent. In some specific conditions, such as liver cirrhosis patients, renal or heart failure patients, thickening of the GB wall can also be mistaken with AC condition [6, 7]. Abdominal CT scan has been shown to have higher sensitivity and specificity in detecting AC. This procedure also can be performed within a short time [8]. However, there are some issues related to this examination, such as radiation exposure, contrast-agent, and unidentified gallstone. A retrospective abdominal CT scan study by Bennet et al. (2001) showed that even though there were 91.7% sensitivity, 99.1% specificity, and 94.3% accuracy in diagnosis AC, however, it showed only 29.3% sensitivity, 96.0% specificity, and 64.1% diagnostic accuracy in EC [9]. In diagnosing acute gangrenous cholecystitis, abdominal CT and trans-abdominal US have low sensitivity. Another imaging, abdominal MRI is considered as a high-level imaging with high sensitivity for biliary system disorders. In AC, not only the increased of signal intensity and thickening of the GB wall signs need to be identified, but also other important factors, such as another possible cause associated with the thickened GB wall, impacted stone at the GB neck or cystic duct, and the GB abnormalities. These parameters' assessment is important assessment before surgery [10, 11]. A prospective study by Hakansson et al. (2000) on diagnostic value comparison between MRI and transabdominal US in patients with suspected of AC revealed that higher sensitivity was found in MRI for diagnosing AC. The MRI sensitivity and specificity were 88% and 89%, whereas it was only 65% and 89% for transabdominal US examination. In MRI based examination, it is easier to detect possible of impacted stone at the cystic duct [12]. Another retrospective study by Fayad et al. (2003) showed that functional method of MRCP increased the diagnostic yield of AC when combined with conventional MRCP method, where the positive predictive value was 100% [13]. In addition, a recent study by Orf et al. (2020) revealed that MRCP could differentiate AC patients with normal CBD caliber, dilated CBD, the cause, and associated anomalies [14]. However, several conditions, such as uncooperative patients, elderly patients, and claustrophobia patients are becoming the major concern.

Endoscopic ultrasound (EUS) is considered to have more advantage in diagnostic view as the probe can be attached to the gastric or duodenal wall providing the closer biliary system images (**Figure 1**) [15]. Etienne et al. reported an emphysematous gallbladder which was successfully diagnosed through EUS procedure, where previous MRCP and contrast CT scan failed to get the diagnosis of AC [16]. It is already known that emphysematous cholecystitis (EC) is AC variant, where it is referring to acute gangrenous cholecystitis which can results in a fatal patient's outcome. The major drawback is that in most of moderate to severe AC cases with

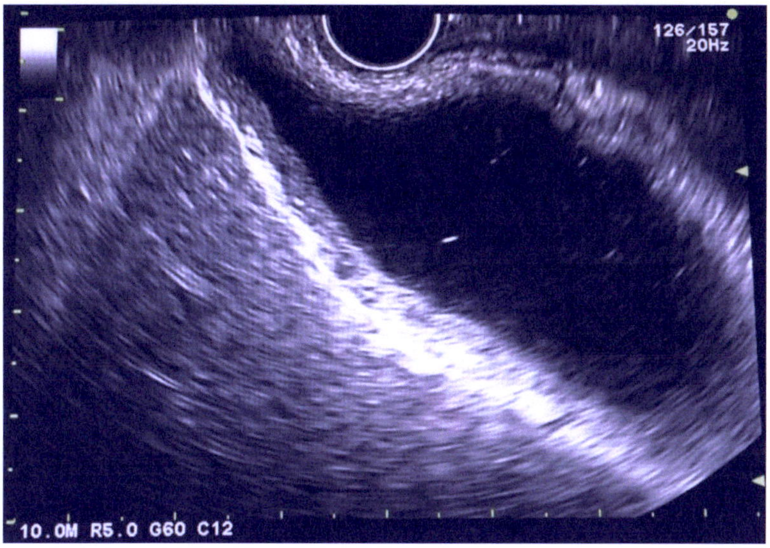

Figure 1.
EUS image showed acute cholecystitis condition. Endoscopy unit Medistra Hospital, Jakarta.

abdominal pain, the commonest diagnostic imaging to be performed is abdominal CT scan [17]. Whereas through MRI examination could have a comprehensive evaluation, including anomaly in biliary system anatomy and the obstructive and non-obstructive common bile duct stones, especially in patients who have experienced acute biliary pancreatitis, however, the cost and long procedure-time issue is still not placing abdominal MRI as the primary modality of choice in acute and severe conditions [18]. EUS has been well-known as an important diagnostic tool for GB abnormalities, stone detection, and especially to confirm the diagnosis of GB carcinoma. A technical review of EUS in GB assessment by Tanaka et al. (2021), it showed how using EUS can get better visualization for complete assessment of gallbladder until the cystic duct by ultrasound probe placement at the gastric anthral area and duodenal bulb [19]. Even though there is no specific paper on how to apply EUS in AC diagnosis, however, the close range of ultrasound probe, the possibility to have complete biliary system evaluation, and the pancreato-biliary connection would give a big advantage in the treatment decision as well as one-stop as well as one-step procedure (diagnostic-therapeutic) in most acute cholecystitis cases with regards to the possibility of surgical approach.

3. The role of interventional EUS in acute cholecystitis

Medical treatment, such as analgesic as well as antibacterial agents, as well as elective or emergency cholecystectomy are still the main recommendation in daily clinical practice with regards to the severity of AC condition. Laparoscopy recently has become the cornerstone in abdominal surgery because of shorter hospital stay, faster wound healing and less pain at surgical incision site. In the severe case, especially two major factors are identified, such as older age (elderly patients) and comorbidity (cardio-pulmonary problems, uncontrolled diabetes mellitus, advance liver and kidney diseases, and critically ill condition), surgical approach might not be performed in the real clinical practice. On the other hand, percutaneous approach (percutaneous transhepatic gallbladder drainage/PTGBD) has become an alternative in such of situations. It is a very easy procedure and can be performed bedside, however, uncooperative patients, altered mental status, risk of infection and catheter dislodgement have raised major concerns [20]. Another method can be performed by ERCP technique by placing nasobiliary tube (NBT) or double pigtail plastic stent into the GB through cystic duct cannulation. Major limitations are normal common bile duct (CBD) cannulation and guide wire insertion to the cystic duct which sometimes is not easy to be performed, especially when there is an obstructed cystic duct [21].

EUS has been used widely for managing biliary disorders, such as EUS-guided biliary drainage (EUS BD) for malignant bile duct obstruction as well as a guide for impacted bile duct stone clearance [22]. In technical review by Rana (2021), the echoendoscope position at duodenal area as the same position where EUS BD is performed, is considered as the best location as it is the nearest location to the GB and cystic duct area. Step by step approach is needed to get the successful result even though sometimes it is not always possible. Stabilizing the scope position is the main key for minimize the complications risk. The next step approach is like EUS BD procedure, puncturing the GB with 19-G FNA needle, bile fluid aspiration, guide wire insertion, then followed by fistula track creation using cautery or non-cautery methods. The most crucial step is the stent delivery and deployed (**Figures 2** and **3**) [23]. A randomized controlled trial between EUS GBD and PTGBD by Jang et al. (2012) showed that both methods have similar technical success rate (97% vs. 97%), and there was not statistically significant in term of complications ($p = .492$) [24]. A systematic review and meta-analysis by Khan et al. (2016) on efficacy and safety of EUS GBD in AC, showing the technical and clinical success rate for transpapillary route was 83% and 93%, whereas transmural route (EUS GBD) technical and clinical success rate were 93% and 97%. The

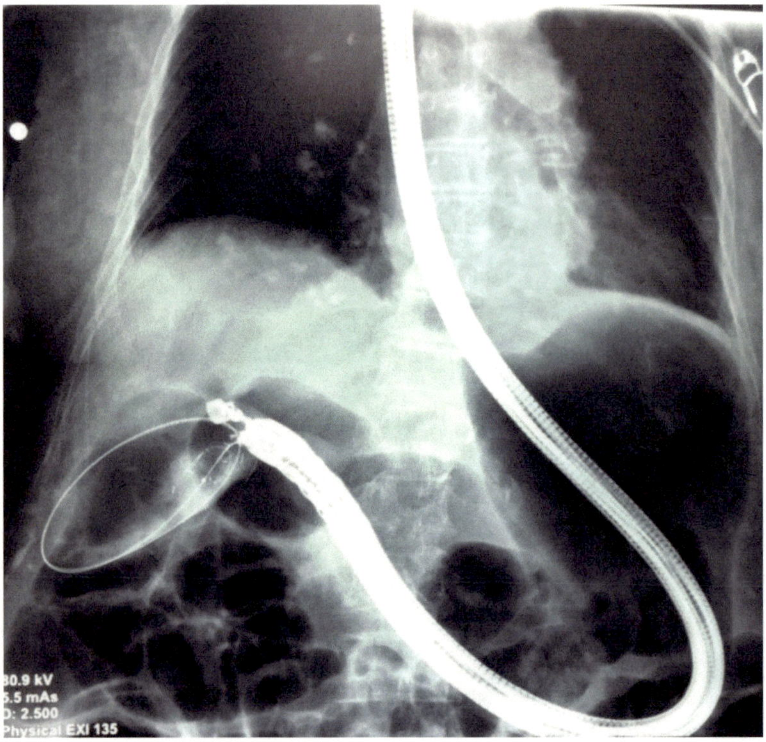

Figure 2.
Fluoroscopy image showed the lumen apposing metallic stent deployment inside the gallbladder. Endoscopy unit Medistra Hospital, Jakarta.

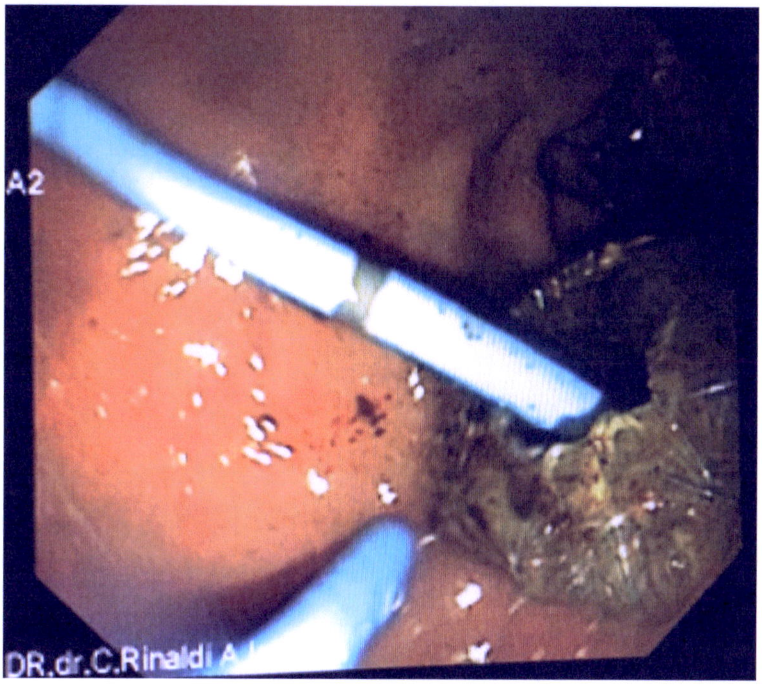

Figure 3.
Endoscopy image of gallbladder drainage with LAMS through the duodenal site. Endoscopy unit, Medistra Hospital, Jakarta.

comparison difference was 10% ($p < .001$) and 4% ($p = .01$). In Endoscopic versus percutaneous methods, recurrent cholecystitis was found more in percutaneous approach than in endoscopic approach [25]. Another study by Tyberg et al. (2016) also shown similar technical success rate between EUS GBD and PTGBD methods [26]. An international multicenter study on EUS GBD in patients who were at high risk for cholecystectomy, showed that the technical and clinical success rate were 95.3%and 90.8%. However, the unplanned events related to the procedure was found higher in non-AC cases than in AC cases with regards to the operator's procedure experience volume [27]. Another retrospective study showed that EUS GBD and percutaneous approach were similarly effective in achieving gallbladder drainage [28]. Recently, there has been a propensity score analysis retrospective study by Teoh et al. (2020) looking at the comparison between EUS GBD and laparoscopic cholecystectomy (LC) for AC, where the result showed the technical success rate was 100% vs. 100%, whereas clinical success rate was 93.3% vs. 100%. After the propensity score matching was done on several factors which might be different from the inclusions' criteria, and there was evidence that two patients died in the EUS GBD group due to aspiration pneumonia and uncontrolled sepsis, however, these events not related to the procedures itself and not statistically significant when compared to the LC group. This study suggested that EUS GBD can be the first approach for patients who are not willing to undergo the surgical approach as well as an alternative in patients who are not fit for surgery. There is no significant difference in the patients' outcome based on 30-day adverse events, recurrent biliary infections, or the need for reintervention [29]. However, there are some major issues which still need to be counted in real clinical practice before it would be recommended in the real clinical practice guideline, such as the cost, operator's experience, multi-disciplinary team approach availability, risk, and complications [30].

4. Conclusions

EUS has a big role in AC condition, where it can be an alternative to patients who are not suitable for surgery. However, a larger study is needed to confirm the previous findings and the patient's long-term outcome. Comprehensive clinical assessment is still the most important thing to do before deciding which is the best method to be performed.

Author details

Cosmas Rinaldi A. Lesmana[1,2*] and Laurentius A. Lesmana[2]

1 Hepatobiliary Division, Department of Internal Medicine, Dr. Cipto Mangunkusumo National General Hospital, Medical Faculty Universitas Indonesia, Jakarta, Indonesia

2 Digestive Disease and Gi Oncology Center, Medistra Hospital, Jakarta, Indonesia

*Address all correspondence to: medicaldr2001id@yahoo.com

References

[1] Indar AA, Beckingham IJ. Acute cholecystitis. BMJ (2002) 325:639-43.

[2] Pisano M, Allievi N, Gurusamy K, Borzellino G, Cimbanassi S, Boerna D, et al. 2020 World society of emergency surgery updated guidelines for the diagnosis and treatment of acute calculus cholecystitis. BMC World J of Emergency Surg (2020) 15:61.

[3] Gomes CA, Junior CS, Di Saveiro S, Sartelli M, Kelly MD, Gomes CC, et al. Acute calculous cholecystitis: review of current best practices. World J Gastrointest Surg (2017) 9(5):118-26.

[4] Okamoto K, Suzuki K, Takada T, Strasberg SM, Asbun HJ, Endo I, et al. Tokyo guidelines 2018: flowchart for the management of acute cholecystitis. J Hepatobiliary Pancreat Sci (2018) 25:55-72.

[5] Kiewiet JJS, Leeuwenburgh MMN, Bipat S, Bossuyt PMM, Stoker J, Boermeester MA. A systematic review and meta-analysis of diagnostic performance of imaging in acute cholecystitis. Radiology (2012) 264:708-20.

[6] Hwang H, Marsh I, Doyle J. Does ultrasonography accurately diagnose acute cholecystitis? Improving diagnostic accuracy based on a review at a regional hospital. Can J Surg (2014) 57:162-8.

[7] Pinto A, Reginelli A, Cagini L, Coppolino F, Ianora AAS, Bracale R, et al. Accuracy of ultrasonohgraphy in the diagnosis of acute calculous cholecystitis: review of the literature. Crit Ultrasound J (2013) 5(Suppl 1):S11.

[8] Schiappacasse G, Soffia P, Silva C, Villacres F. Computed tomography imaging of complications of acute cholecystitis. Indian J Radiol Imaging (2018) 28:195-9.

[9] Bennet GL, Rusinek H, Lisi V, Israel GM, Krinsky GA, Slywotzky CM, et al. CT findings in acute gangrenous cholecystitis. AJR (2002) 178:275-81.

[10] Watanabe Y, Nagayama M, Okumura A, Amoh Y, Katsube T, Suga T, et al. MR imaging of acute biliary disorders. RadioGraphics (2007) 27:477-95.

[11] Catalano OA, Sahani DV, Kalva SP, Cushing MS, Hahn PF, Brown JJ, et al. MR imaging of the gallbladder: a pictorial essay. RadioGraphics (2008) 28:135-55.

[12] Hakansson K, Leander P, Ekberg O, Hakansson HO. MR imaging in clinically suspected acute cholecystitis. Act Radiol (2000) 41:322-8.

[13] Fayad LM, Holland GA, Bergin D, Iqbal N, Parker L, Curcillo PG, et al. Functional magnetic resonance cholangiography (fMRC) of the gallbladder and biliary tree with contrast-enhanced magnetic resonance cholangiography. J of magnetic resonance imaging (2003) 18:449-60.

[14] Orf AA, Waheed KB, Alshehri AS, Algarni MA, Altaf B, Amjad M, et al. Magnetic resonance cholangio-pancreatography in patients with acute cholecystitis and cholestatic liver pattern – what to expect? J Evolution Med Dent Sci (2020) 9:2436-441.

[15] Chantarojanasiri T, Hirooka Y, Kawashima H, Ohno E, Kongkam P, Goto H. The role of endoscopic ultrasound in the diagnosis of gallbladder diseases. J Med Ultrasonics (2017) 44:63-70.

[16] Etienne D, Sharma S, Changela K, Duddempudi S. A curious case of emphysematous gallbladder and the diagnostic role of endoscopic

ultrasound. Am J Gastroenterol (2017) 112:p S695.

[17] Safwan M, Penny SM. Emphysematous cholecystitis: a deadly twist to a common disease. J of Diag Med Sonograph (2016) 32:131-7.

[18] Murphy MC, Gibney B, Gillespie C, Hynes J, Bolster F. Gallstones top to toe: what the radiologist needs to know. Insight into imaging (2020) 11:13.

[19] Tanaka K, Katanuma A, Hayashi T, Kin T, Takahashi K. Roel of endoscopic ultrasound for gallbladder disease. J of Med Ultrasonics (2021) 48:187-98.

[20] Mou D, Tesfasilassie T, Hirji S, Ashley SW. Advances in the management of acute cholecystitis. Ann Gastroenterol Surg (2019) 3:247-53.

[21] Sobani ZA, Ling C, Rustagi T. Endoscopic transpapillary gallbladder drainage for acute cholecystitis. Dig Dis Sci (2021) 66:1425-35.

[22] Lesmana CRA, Mandasari BKD. The new era of endoscopic ultrasound in biliary disorders. Clin J Gastroenterol (2021) DOI: 10.1007//s12328-021-01419-1.

[23] Rana SS. Endoscopic ultrasound-guided gallbladder drainage: a technical review. Ann of Gastroenterol (2021) 34:1-7.

[24] Jang JW, Lee SS, Song TJ, Hyun YS, Park DH, Seo DW, et al. Endoscopic ultrasound-guided transmural and percutaneous transhepatic gallbladder drainage are comparable for acute cholecystitis. Gastroenterol (2012) 142:805-11.

[25] Khan MA, Atiq O, Kubiliun N, Ali B, Kamal F, Nollan R, et al. Efficacy and safety of endoscopic gallbladder drainage in acute cholecystitis: is it better than percutaneous gallbladder drainage? A systematic review and meta-analysis. Gastrointest Endosc (2016) DOI: 10.1016/j.gie.2016.06.032.

[26] Tyberg A, Saumoy M, Sequeiros EV, Giovannini M, Artifon E, Teoh A, et al. EUS-guided versus percutaneous gallbladder drainage isn't it time to convert? J of Clin Gastroenterol (2016) DOI: 10.1097/MCG.0000000000000786.

[27] Teoh AY, Miranda MP, Kunda R, Lee SS, Irani S, Yeaton P, et al. Outcomes of an international multicenter registry on EUS-guided gallbladder drainage in patients at high risk for cholecystectomy. Endosc Int Open (2019) 07:E964-E973.

[28] Teoh AYB, Serna C, Penas I, Chong CCN, Miranda MP, Ng EKW, et al. Endoscopic ultrasound-guided gallbladder drainage reduces adverse events compared with percutaneous cholecystostomy in patients who are unfit for cholecystectomy.

[29] Teoh AYB, Leung CH, Tam PTH, Yeung KKYA, Mok RCY, Chan DL, et al. EUS-guided gallbladder drainage versus laparoscopic cholecystectomy for acute cholecystitis: a propensity score analysis with 1-year follow up data. Gastrointest Endosc (2020) http://doi.org/10.1016/j.gie.2020.

[30] Posner H, Widmer J. EUSguided gallbladder drainage. Transl Gastroenterol Hepatol (2020) 5:41.

Chapter 6

Acute Alitasic Cholecystitis

Giovanni Petracca, Francesco Zappia, Maccarone Giuseppe, Mazzeo Mariano, Mio Francesco, Fabrizio Silvaggio, Mileto Ivana, Plutino Francesco, Posterino Antonietta and Danilo Cafaro

Abstract

Acute acalculous cholecystitis (AAC) is the inflammatory disease of the gallbladder in the absence of gallstones. Typically affects critically ill patients. Diagnosis is not straightforward as Murphy's sign is difficult to detect in critically ill and many imaging findings are numb or nonspecific. Acalculous cholecystitis is a life-threatening disorder that has a high risk of perforation and necrosis compared to the more typical calculous disease. Management involves a percutaneous cholecystostomy, a surgical cholecystectomy, or, more recently, a metal stent placed endoscopically through the gastrointestinal tract into the gallbladder. Acalculous cholecystitis is a serious illness that has high morbidity and mortality. The reported mortality of the condition varies from 30 to 50% depending on the age of the patient. Even those who survive have a long recovery that can take months.

Keywords: cholecystitis, gallbladder, alithiasic

1. Introduction

Acute alithiasic cholecystitis is defined as an inflammatory disease of the gallbladder in the absence of gallstones or obstruction of the cystic duct and it has a multifactorial pathogenesis [1].

It accounts for approximately 10% (range, 2% -15%) of all cases of acute cholecystitis. Acute alithisiac cholecystitis occurs in approximately 0.2% -0.4% of all critically ill patients. Duncan recognized it, for the first time, in 1844 when a fatal case of acute cholecystitis complicating an incarcerated hernia was reported [2]. Acute cholecystitis acalculous is associated with a morbidity more serious and a rate mortality more elevated compared to acute lithiasic cholecystitis [3].

The death rate depends primarily on the presentation already critical of the patient as the disease affects both medically and surgically compromised patients. Clinically, acute alithiasic cholecystitis is indistinguishable from acute lithiasic cholecystitis. Many patients with acute cholecystitis acalculous have the same symptoms of gallstone cholecystitis: pain in the quadrant abdominal upper right, fever, neutrophili leukocytosis, elevated liver enzymes (ALT, AST, Alkaline phosphatase) increased serum total bilirubinand fractional [4].

There are various risk factors that predispose to the formation of acute alithiasic cholecystitis which are listed in **Table 1**, as noted this pathology mainly

Risk factors commonly associated with acute alithiasic cholecystitis	Risk factors rarely associated with acute alithiasic cholecystitis
Severe trauma leading to hospitalization; some factors particularly useful for the diagnosis of acute alithiasic cholecystitis are blood transfusions (over 12 units) and cardiac arrhythmias.	Hypovolemia
Recent cardio-pulmonary surgery	Cholangiopancreatography Endoscopic retrograde
Shock of any kind	Longer of hospital stay
Severe burns	Immunodeficiency: acquired immunodeficiency syndrome, organ transplant
Bacterial or viral sepsis	Chronic disease: diabetes, hypertension, atherosclerotic disease, morbid obesity
Critical illness (any patient requiring mechanical ventilation in the ICU)	Vasculitis: Churg- Strauss, giant cell arteritis, Henoch-Shonlein purpura, polyartereitis nodosa, lupus.
Total parenteral nutrition	
Prolonged fasting	

Owen & Jain [5] table.

Table 1.
Descending order of risk factors associated with acute alithiasic cholecystitis.

affects patients in serious clinical conditions: severe trauma, patients with shock of any type on mechanical ventilation, with sepsis, burns or in total parenteral nutrition [6].

2. Pathophysiology

The etiology of acute cholecystitis acalculous is multifactorial, but is mainly formed by biliary stasis or organ wall ischemia. Biliary stasis can be caused by fasting, post-surgical total parenteral nutrition that leads to an increase in bile viscosity which irritates the mucous membrane of the gallbladder. Gallbladder wall ischemia occurs due to decreased blood flow due to fever, dehydration, or heart failure, which leads to the pathogenesis of acute cholecystitis [7].

It arises acutely when the walls of the gallbladder become inflamed for the reasons mentioned above [8].

Prolonged ischemia of the gallbladder walls leads to gangrene and then perforation. If the process occurs slowly, the formation of cholecystoduodenal (70%), cholecystocholic (10–20%), and the less common cholecystogastric fistula is possible. This will lead to sepsis and shock. These findings are referred to as acute cholecystitis. Chronic acalculous cholecystitis usually presents more insidiously. Symptoms are more prolonged and may be less severe. Symptoms may also be more intermittent and vague, although patients can present with signs of acute biliary colic [9].

3. Epidemiology

Acalculous cholecystitis has an incidence rate of 0.12% in the entire population.

Rates are increased in HIV and other immunosuppressed patients. These individuals are more susceptible to certain opportunistic infections such as microsporidia, cytomegalovirus (CMV), and Cryptosporidium, which can seed and flourish in bile within the gallbladder [10].

Carriers of *G. lamblia*, *H. pylori*, and *S. typhi* are also associated with increased risks to develop cholecystitis.

It can occur in all breeds. Acute alithiasic cholecystitis has a slight male predominance (80% of case), unlike acute lithiasic cholecystitis, which has a female predominance and occurs at any age with a criticality threshold between the fourth and eighth decade of life [11].

4. Prognosis

Acalculous cholecystitis is a serious illness that has high morbidity and mortality. The reported mortality of the condition varies from 30 to 50% depending on the age of the patient. Even those who survive have a long recovery that can take months [12].

5. Mortality/morbidity

The rates of the mortality and morbidity associated with acute cholecystitis can be high; the disease is frequently seen in patients with sepsis or other serious conditions. The reported mortality range is 10% - 50% for acute cholecystitis acalculous compared to 1% for acute cholecystitis lithiasic [13].

6. Complications

Perforations or gangrene of the gallbladder and exstrabiliary abscess formation in the acute alithiasic versus lithiasic gallbladder may occur [14].

7. History and physical Exam

Often these patients are very seriously admitted to intensive care in mechanical ventilation and cannot participate in an anamnestic interview and therefore communicate their symptoms. Physical examination may detect fever, tenderness on the upper abdominal quadrants of the right associated with laboratory abnormalities such as neutrophil leukocytosis and altered liver tests (high values for ALT, AST, alkaline phosphatase and direct bilirubin) [15].

8. Diagnosis

The diagnosis of acute cholecystitis acalculous is difficult because no clinical data (symptoms, examination goal, testing laboratory) establish it. Although no combination of clinical factors will lead to the diagnosis, there seems to be a consensus on the fact that a high clinical suspicion for acute cholecystitis acalculous is indicated in all critically ill patients for whom no etiology has been found. The final diagnosis of acute cholecystitis is mainly based on radiological and ultrasound findings [16–18].

9. Radiology

There is controversy about what is the best imaging modality and which to use in the diagnosis of cholecystitis acute acalculous. However, radiological criteria for the

Mode	Criteria	Diagnosis
Abdominal ultrasound	Major: 3.5- to 4-mm (or more) thick wall (if at least 5-cm distended longitudinally with no ascites or hypoalbuminemia) Pericholecystic fluid (halo)/subserosal edema Intramural gas Sloughed mucosal membrane	2 major or 1 major and 2 minor (most studies have favored the diagnostic triad—wall thickness, sludge, hydrops)
	Minors: Echogenic bile (sludge) Hydrops distension greater than 8-cm longitudinally or 5-cm transversely (with clear fluid)	
TC	Major: 3- to 4-mm wall thickness Pericholecystic fluid Subserosal edema Intramural gas Sloughed mucosa	2 major or 1 major and 2 minor
	Minors: Hyperdense bile (sludge) Subjective distension (hydrops)	

Table 2.
Imaging criteria.

diagnosis of acute alithic cholecystitis have been developed for the use of ultrasound and computed tomography. MRI is not used because it is a lengthy procedure with no benefit compared to the other modalities [19]. CT offers few advantages over ultrasound abdominal, unless there are other intra-abdominal pathologies that cannot be studied with the ultrasound. Therefore, abdominal ultrasound was the first line for the diagnosis of acute alithiasic cholecystitis as it can be performed at the bedside and favors patients who are intrasportable [20]. The ultrasound criteria for diagnosing acute alithiasic cholecystitis are: the thickness of the gallbladder wall, dangerous cystic fluid, wall, edema intramural gas, desquamated mucosa, mud or hydrops. The thickness of the gallbladder wall (3.5–4 mm) has been considered a crucial component for the diagnosis of acute alithiasic cholecystitis. Therefore, abdominal ultrasound is a very useful tool for diagnosing acute alithiasic cholecystitis as many prospective studies have suggested and, also, it is easy to use, fast, portable and easily repeatable at the bedside [21–23].

CT is useful for diagnosing acute alithiasic cholecystitis and other abdominal diseases. it requires patient transport, which may not be feasible, and offers few advantages compared to abdominal ultrasound. However, with a normal ultrasound, CT can diagnose acute alithiasic cholecystitis and make a differential diagnosis (**Table 2**) [5, 24, 25].

10. Therapy

The two prevalent treatment options for acute alithiasic cholecystitis are cholecystostomy (gallbladder drainage) and/or cholecystectomy. Other methods such as ERCP using stents or tubes have been tried but unsuccessful. Cholecystectomy is generally considered the definitive therapy. Some authors propose cholecystostomy as the only treatment. Others claim that the cholecystostomy is just a bridge to the cholecystectomy more secure or just a treatment to see if the acute cholecystitis acalculous is resolved. Therefore, Boland et al. recommend the cholecystostomy prophylactic for all intensive care patients with abdominal sepsis who do not improve with medical therapy (high-dose antibiotic therapy) [26, 27].

The cholecystostomy is generrally plausible, quick and safe; it can be performed transperitoneally or transhepatically under ultrasound or CT guidance by interventional surgeons or radiologists. Therefore, cholecystostomy can provide time to optimize the patient's condition for cholecystectomy surgery. There seems to be an unanimous tendency to favor the cholecystostomy before cholecystectomy, unless there is a strong evidence of an ischemic cholecystitis that the drainage alone does not alleviate.

Cholecystectomy is a definitive therapy when performed by open or laparoscopic surgery. Laparoscopic surgery has been favored in recent years because it can be both diagnostic and therapeutic, it is less invasive, and it has similar morbidity and mortality compared to open procedures [28–31]. However, it should be noted that it may need to be converted to an open cholecystectomy and this should not be considered a failure of the surgeon on the contrary, when faced with situations in which it is not possible to distinguish, due to the inflammatory state of the gallbladder, the various structures anatomical, conversion to "open surgery" is preferable [32–35].

11. Conclusions

When an acalculous acute cholecystitis is suspected, the cholecystostomy must be carried out immediately, because the patient can only improve with this technique. If the improvement occurs with the decompression and drainage through cholecystostomy, the tube can be removed after 3 weeks, and this is the only treatment needed [36–39]. If there is no improvement, urgent cholecystectomy should be strongly considered as it can save the patient's life and thus improve abdominal sepsis [40–42].

Author details

Giovanni Petracca*, Francesco Zappia, Maccarone Giuseppe, Mazzeo Mariano, Mio Francesco, Fabrizio Silvaggio, Mileto Ivana, Plutino Francesco, Posterino Antonietta and Danilo Cafaro
Azienda Sanitaria Provinciale di Vibo Valentia, Italy

*Address all correspondence to: doc37@virgilio.it

References

[1] Treinen C, Lomelin D, Krause C, Goede M, Oleynikov D.Colecistite acuta acuta nei malati critici: fattori di rischio e strategie chirurgiche. *Langenbecks Arch Surg*. 2015 maggio. 400 (4): 421-7. [Medline].

[2] The Management of Gallstone Disease: A Practical and Evidence-Based Approach a cura di Michael R. Cox, Guy D. Eslick, Robert Padbury.

[3] Tana M, Tana C, Cocco G, Iannetti G, Romano M, Schiavone C.Colecistite acuta acuta e malattie cardiovascolari: terra di confusione. *J Ultrasound*. 18 dicembre 2015 (4): 317-20. [Medline].

[4] Theodorou P, Maurer CA, Spanholtz TA, et al. Colecistite acuta in pazienti gravemente ustionati: incidenza e fattori predisponenti. *Ustioni*. 2009 maggio. 35 (3): 405-11. [Medline].

[5] Laurila J, Laurila PA, Saarnio J, et al. Organ system dysfunction following open cholecystectomy for acute acalculous cholecystitis in critically ill patients. Acta Anaesthesiol Scand 2006;50: 173-179.Laurila JJ, Ala-Kokko TI, Laurila PA, et al. Histopathology of acute acalculous cholecystitis in critically ill patients. Histopathology 2005;47:485-492.

[6] Hamp T, Fridrich P, Mauritz W, Hamid L, Pelinka LE. Colecistite dopo un trauma. *J Trauma*. 2009 febbraio 66 (2): 400-6. [Medline].

[7] Basar O, Kisacik B, Bozdogan E, et al. Una causa insolita di colecistite acuta durante la gravidanza: il virus dell'epatite A. *Dig Dis Sci*. 50 agosto 2005 (8): 1532. [Medline].

[8] Fuoti M, Pinotti M, Miceli V, et al. [Colecistite acuta acuta come complicanza dell'epatite A: rapporto di 2 casi pediatrici] [Italiano]. *Pediatr Med Chir*. 2008 marzo-aprile. 30 (2): 102-5. [Medline].

[9] Inagaki FF, Hara Y, Kamei M, Tanaka M, Yasuno M. Colecistite acuta e cronica acuta associata a dissezione aortica. *Rappresentante del caso J Surg*. 2015 1 agosto 2015 (8): [Medline]. [Testo completo].

[10] Gu MG, Kim TN, Song J, Nam YJ, Lee JY, Park JS. Fattori di rischio e risultati terapeutici della colecistite acuta acuta. *Digestione*. 2014. 90 (2): 75-80. [Medline].

[11] Wood BE, Trautman J, Smith N, Putnis S. Caso clinico raro di colecistite acuta: torsione della cistifellea con conseguente rottura. *SAGE Open Med Case Rep*. 2019. 7: 2050313X18823385. [Medline]. [Testo completo].

[12] Joseph T, Unver K, Hwang GL, et al. Colecistostomia percutanea per colecistite acuta: esperienza decennale. *J Vasc Interv Radiol*. 23 gennaio 2012 (1): 83-8.e1. [Medline].

[13] Chung YH, Choi ER, Kim KM, et al. La colecistostomia percutanea può essere una gestione definitiva per la colecistite acuta acuta ?. *J Clin Gastroenterol*. 46 marzo 2012 (3): 216-9. [Medline].

[14] Noh SY, Gwon DI, Ko GY, Yoon HK, Sung KB. Ruolo della colecistostomia percutanea per la colecistite acuta acuta: risultati clinici di 271 pazienti. *Eur Radiol*. 28 aprile 2018 (4): 1449-55. [Medline].

[15] Soria Aledo V, Galindo Iniguez L, Flores Funes D, Carrasco Prats M, Aguayo Albasini JL. La colecistectomia è il trattamento di scelta per la colecistite acuta acuta? Una revisione sistematica della letteratura. *Rev Esp Enferm Dig*. 109 ottobre 2017 (10): 708-18. [Medline]. [Testo completo].

[16] Kirkegard J, Horn T, Christensen SD, Larsen LP, Knudsen AR, Mortensen FV. La colecistostomia percutanea è

un'opzione di trattamento definitivo efficace per la colecistite acuta acuta. *Scand J Surg*. 104 dicembre 2015 (4): 238-43. [Medline].

[17] Irani S, Baron TH, Grimm IS, Khashab MA. Drenaggio della cistifellea guidato dall'EUS con uno stent metallico che appoggia il lume (con video). *Gastrointest Endosc*. 2015 dicembre 82 (6): 1110-5. [Medline].

[18] Casillas RA, Yegiyants S, Collins JC. La colecistectomia laparoscopica precoce è la gestione preferita della colecistite acuta. *Arch Surg*. 2008 giugno 143 (6): 533-7. [Medline].

[19] Schuld J, Glanemann M. Colecistite acuta. *Viszeralmedizin*. 31 giugno 2015 (3): 163-5. [Medline].

[20] Anderson JE, Inui T, Talamini MA, Chang DC. La colecistostomia non offre alcun beneficio in termini di sopravvivenza nei pazienti con colecistite acuta acuta e sepsi e shock gravi. *J Surg Res*. 190 agosto 2014 (2): 517-21. [Medline].

[21] Jones MW, Ferguson T.Colecistite acuta. *StatPearls [Internet]*. 16 gennaio 2019. 2018: [Medline]. [Testo completo].

[22] Barie PS, Eachempati SR. Acute acalculous cholecystitis. Curr Gastroenterol Rep 2003;5:302-309.

[23] Owen CC, Jain R. Acute acalculous cholecystitis. Curr Treat Options Gastroenterol 2005;8:99-104.

[24] Beckman I, Dash N, Sefczek RJ, et al. Ultrasonographic findings in acute acalculous cholecystitis. Gastrointest Radiol 1985;10 387-389.

[25] Mariat G, Mahul P, Prev TN, et al. Contribution of ultrasonography and cholescintigraphy to the diagnosis of acute acalculous cholecystitis in intensive care unit patients. Intensive Care Med 2000;26:1658-1663.

[26] Boland GW, Slater G, Lu DS, et al. Prevalence and significance of gallbladder abnormalities seen on sonography in intensive care unit patients. *AJR Am J Roentgenol*. 2000;174(4):973-7.

[27] Ryu JK, Ryu KH, Kim KH. Clinical features of acute acalculous cholecystitis. J Clin Gastroenterol 2003;36:166-169.

[28] Glenn F, Becker CG. Acute acalculous cholecystitis. An increasing entity. Ann Surg 1982;195:131-136.

[29] Inoue T, Mishima Y. Postoperative acute cholecystitis: a collective review of 494 cases in Japan. Jpn J Surg 1988;18: 35-42.

[30] McChesney JA, Northup PG, Bickston SJ. Acute acalculous cholecystitis associated with systemic sepsis and visceral arterial hypoperfusion: a case series and review of pathophysiology. Dig Dis Sci 2003;48:1960-1967.Wang AJ, Wang TE, Lin CC, et al. Clinical predictors of severe gallbladder complications in acute acalculous cholecystitis. World J Gastroenterol 2003;9:2821-2823.

[31] Kalliafas S, Ziegler DW, Flancbaum L, et al. Acute acalculous cholecystitis: incidence, risk factors, diagnosis, and outcome. Am Surg 1998;64:471-475.

[32] Deitch EA, Engel JM. Ultrasonic detection of acute cholecystitis with pericholecystic abscesses. Am Surg 1981;47:211-214.

[33] Yasuda H, Takada T, Kawarada Y, et al. Unusual cases of acute cholecystitis and cholangitis: Tokyo guidelines. J Hepatobiliary Pancreat 2007;14:98-113.

[34] Westlake PJ, Hershfiled NB, Kelly JK, et al. Chronic right upper quadrant pain without gallstones: does

HIDA scan predict outcome after cholecystectomy? Am J Gastroenterol 1990;85:986– 990.

[35] Ziessman HA. Cholecystokinin cholescintigraphy: clinical indications and proper methodology. Update Nucl Med 2001;39:997-1006.Shuman WP, Rogers JV, Rudd TG, et al. Low sensitivity of sonography and cholescintigraphy in acalculous cholecystitis. AJR Am J Roentgenol 1984;142:531-534.

[36] Taoka H. Experimental study on the pathogenesis of acute acalculous cholecystitis, with special reference to the roles of microcirculatory disturbances, free radicals and membrane-bound phospholipase A2. Gastroenterol Jpn 1991;26:633-644.

[37] Sanda RB. Acute acalculous cholecystitis after trauma: the role of microcirculatory failure and cellular hypoxia. South Med J 2008;101: 1087-1088.

[38] Hakala T, Nuutinen PJ, Ruokonen ET, et al. Microangiopathy in acute acalculous cholecystitis. Br J Surg 1997;84:1249-1252.

[39] Mirvis SE, Vainright JR, Nelson AW, et al. The diagnosis of acute acalculous cholecystitis: a comparison of sonography, scintigraphy, and CT. AJR Am J Roentgenol 1986;147:1171-1175.

[40] Boland GWL, Slater G, Lu DSK, et al. Prevalence and significance of gallbladder abnormalities seen on sonography in intensive care unit patients. AJR Am J Roentgenol 2000;174:973-977.

[41] Deitch EA, Engel JM. Acute acalculous cholecystitis. Ultrasonic diagnosis. Am J Surg 1981;142:290-292.

[42] Deitch EJM. Ultrasound in elective biliary tract surgery. Am J Surg 1980;140:277-283.

Chapter 7

Pathophysiology of Gallstones

Mela Ram Attri, Irshad Ahmad Kumar, Ferkhand Mohi Ud Din, Ashiq Hussain Raina and Aakarshit Attri

Abstract

Gallstones are the stones developing in the gallbladder. Evolution of pathophysiology changes the trends of treatment of a disease. Laparoscopic revolution was only because of gallstones diseases. The shifting of food habits increased the incidence of diseases in developing countries. There are mainly three types of stones Cholesterol, pigment and brown stones. The pathophysiology of which is different for each type. Cholesterol stones being most common owing to the risk factors being prevalent in the developing and developed societies. Pigment stones being most common in blood disorder patients while brown stones are most common in common bile duct and are infected ones.

Keywords: gallstone, pathogenesis, cholesterol, pigment stones, diet, genes

1. Introduction

The gallstones (**Figure 1**) are hard, pebble-like pieces of material, usually made of cholesterol or bilirubin, that develop in the gallbladder [1]. These stones are formed due to various disorders. Five defects primarily play critical role in pathogenesis of cholesterol stones Viz lithogenes and genetic factors; hepatic hypersecretion of cholesterol; rapid phase transition of cholesterol in bile; impaired gallbladder motility; intestinal factors involving absorption of cholesterol, slow intestinal motility and altered gut microbiota.

Gallstones affect about 15% of United States population. About 10–20% of the United States population will get gallstones at some point in their life time and females are more affected than men [2].

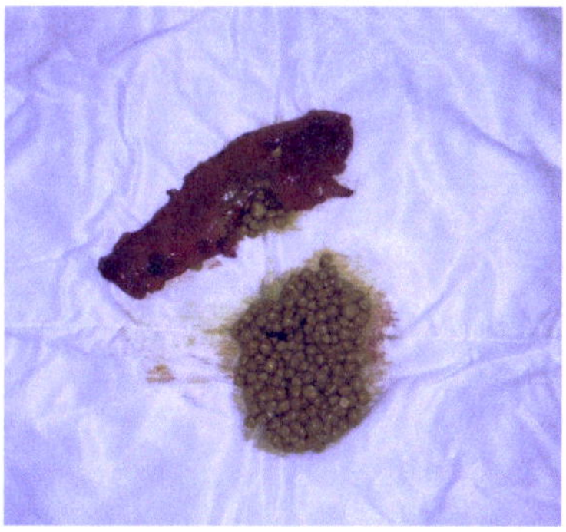

Figure 1.
Cholesterol gallstones and gallbladder after cholecystectomy.

Gallstones can cause biliary colic, cholecystitis, pancreatitis, empyema Gallbladder, perforation of gallbladder, cholangitis, bile duct obstruction [3], and cancers (gallbladder [4], colorectal [5, 6], pancreatic [7]). In 85% of patients with gallbladder cancer, gall stones are present [8]. Gallbladder cancer is a very fatal cancer with average survival of 6 months [9] and 5-year survival rate of 5% [8]. This bad prognosis is because of silent features. An increased mortality from cardiovascular disease and cancer was found to be associated with gallstones by an 18 year national study [10]. Asymptomatic cholelithiasis are present in 80% of cases and most of these are incidentally found when the patients are under investigation for other ailments [11]. In general, 10–25% of asymptomatic cases may develop symptoms during the patient's lifetime [12]. The estimated cost for gallbladder diseases was 6.5 billion dollar annually in United States only in 2002 [13].

There are three types of gallstones; first and most common type is cholesterol stone. Black and brown pigmented stones are the other two types of gallstones. The prevalence of various types of gallstones in the western world is: 75% of gallstones are cholesterol stones, 20% are black pigment stones, and 5% or less are brown pigment stones. Cholesterol and black pigment stones are formed exclusively in gallbladder in a sterile medium, while as brown pigment stones are formed everywhere in the biliary tree owing to the anaerobic bacterial infection. Stasis of bile is an essential component in the formation of gallstone or bile duct stone formation [14]. In underdeveloped countries parasitic infection of biliary tree is associated with brown pigment stones [15].

Physical-chemical origin is the basis of pathogenesis of sterile stones (cholesterol and black pigment stones) [16]. There is an alteration in lipid and lipo-pigment composition which results in the formation of stones. In cholesterol and black pigment stones the major component is cholesterol monohydrate crystals and calcium hydrogen bilirubinate respectively. During the long stay in gallbladder, the black pigment gets degraded and polymerized by free radicals and helps in the formation of black pigment stones while as in the brown pigment stones the main mechanism is infectious where the enzymatic hydrolysis of biliary lipids by anaerobic bacterial enzymes produces supersaturated long chain fatty and deconjugated bile acids [14, 17].

2. Risk factors

Gallstone formation occurs as a result of interaction between genetic and environmental factors in which few are unmodifiable and unaltered as age and genetic makeup. The traditional risk factors for gallstones are four "F" female, fertile, fat, forty and some have added fifth "F" for fair skin [18].

Various intrinsic and extrinsic risk factors for the causation of different types of gallstones are genetic factors, advanced age, female gender, parity, ethnicity, rapid weight loss, different medications (oestrogen replacement therapy, oral contraceptive pills), total parenteral nutrition [19], obesity, westernized diet, Type 2 diabetes mellitus, metabolic syndrome [20], dyslipidaemia, hyperinsulinemia [21], increased enterohepatic circulation of bilirubin [22], defective gall bladder motility [23] as shown in **Table 1**.

2.1 Age and genetics

Age is an important factor for the stone formation, with increase in age enzyme 7 α hydroxylase (Limiting enzyme for bile acid synthesis) activity decreases which increases the saturation of cholesterol in bile and hence increasing the chances of stone formation [24].

Risk factors for gallstone diseases	
Intrinsic factor	**Extrinsic factor**
Age	Lipid profile
Gender	Diet
Ethnicity	Obesity
Defective gallbladder motility	Weight loss
	Physical activity
Genetics	Diseases
	Medication

Table 1.
Risk factors for gallbladder stone diseases.

Various genes are linked with increased susceptibility of gallstones like Lith genes identified in mouse models [25]. Two variants of ATP binding Cassette transporters ABCG5-R50C and ABCG8-D19H [26]; 3 variants of Farnesoid X Receptor gene (FXR) (rs 35724, rs 11110358, rs 11110386) [27]; polymorphism of apolipoprotein E4 allele [28]; mucin genes [29]; fibroblast growth factor receptor 4 (FGFR4) [30], polymorphism in CCK 1-R gene [31] are linked with cholelithiasis. The genetic factors are responsible for 25–30% of symptomatic gallstones as inferred from twin studies [32]. Gene expressions are affected by environmental factors and gene-environmental interactions through epigenetic mechanisms [33] also involving fat storage and insulin resistance [34]. These factors primarily include micro RNAs [35] Viz. 114 miRNA [36], miR-122 [37].

2.2 Gender and ethnicity

Females are having a higher risk factors due to various reasons for cholelithiasis such as higher oestrogen levels naturally [38], multiparity [39] and ingestion of oral contraceptives containing oestrogens [38]. Females also tend to undergo cholecystectomy procedure more than males [40].

Ethnicity plays an important non-modifiable role in cholelithiasis as few ethnic groups are having higher incidence of having gall stones as in North American Indians (73% among women more than 30 years old within Prima Tribe) [14], American Indians (men 29.5%, women 64.1%) [41]. Prevalence of Gallstone and Gallbladder Cancer are co-related and effects certain indigenous population like South America & North India, especially younger population [42].

Risk of deaths from gallbladder cancer and other malignancies has been observed to be seven times more in tribal members with gallstones [43].

2.3 Lipid profile and diet

The co-relation between lipids and cholesterol stone formation is complex, multi factorial and is dependent on other factors also as few studies are in favour and few showing inverse relationship [14]. Few studies show high LDL [44], high cholesterol [45], low HDL [46] are associated with higher gall stone formation which seems to be evident but other studies show there are having inverse relationship with gallstone formation like low HDL, high cholesterol and high LDL [14].

Cholesterol gallstones are associated with western diet [47]. Multiple studies have shown high carbohydrate intake couples with high glycemic load [48], chronic hypernutrition [49] fibre depleted diet [50] are associated with higher risk for cholelithiasis in process which are associated with decreased risk are intake of in saturated fat [51], coffee [52], fibre [53], fish oil [54], calcium [55], ascorbic acid [56], fresh fruits and vegetables [57] and nuts [51].

2.4 Obesity and weight loss

Obesity is itself risk factor for cholelithiasis. It has been shown that an obese women (BMI $\geq$ 30 kg/m^2) has two fold and morbidly obese women (BMI $\geq$ 45 kg/m^2) has seven fold higher risk for cholelithiasis as compared to lean women (BMI < 25 kg/m^2) [58].

Rapid weight loss i.e., >1.5 kg/week and or loss of body weight >25% [59] are risk factors for cholelithiasis which usually occur after bariatric surgery. Weight loss has also been found to reduce risk of gallstones except when rapid loss occurs.

2.5 Physical activity

Physical activity decreases risk for cholelithiasis [60] as it improves hepatobiliary funtions, gut motility [61], increasing HDL [62], improves insulin release and plasma triglyceride levels [63]. An endurance exercise (cycling and running) 5 times per week for 30 minutes daily decreases risk by 34% for cholelithiasis [64] or 2–3 h/week of recreational exercise decrease risk by 20% for cholecystectomy [60]. While as reduced physical activity increases risk for cholelithiasis [64].

2.6 Diseases

Various diseases increase the risk for cholelithiasis as these work by different mechanisms like causing abnormal gallbladder motility, malabsorption of bile salts, decreased bile salt synthesis [65], increasing bile cholesterol saturation [66], supersaturation of bile and increased hepatic cholesterol secretion [67]. Different diseases increasing risk for cholelithiasis viz. metabolic syndrome, dyslipidaemia, diabetes (2–3 fold [68]), insulin resistance or hyperinsulinemia [69], chronic hepatitis C virus [66], liver cirrhosis (25–30% increased risk [65] and Chron's disease [70].

2.7 Alcohol and smoking

Both these habits have controversial results from various studies some favouring and others refuting association with cholelithiasis.

Men consuming alcohol 0–20 g per day have higher risk than those who consume 20–60 g per day [24]. But few studies show severe alcohol abuse in itself and also led to chronic cirrhosis (pigment stones), which is an independent risk factor for cholelithiasis [71].

Cigarette smoking is another risk factor for gallstones among woman [72], while as few studies refute these claims show no association with gallstones [73].

2.8 Intestinal absorption of cholesterol

An imbalance between absorption and synthesis of cholesterol i.e., increased biliary cholesterol secretion from high dietary cholesterol and decreased bile acid synthesis and pool, all driving bile supersaturation [22]. High cholesterol diet and high intestinal cholesterol absorption are two independent risk factors for gallstones [74], regulated by many factors like expression of sterol transport protein [75].

2.9 Gut microbiota

In patients with cholelithiasis there is evidence of altered gut microbiota with increment of intestinal bacterial phylum proteobacteria decrement of *Faecalibacterium* spp., *Lechnospira* spp., and *Roseburia* spp. [76], also increased amount of Gam positive anaerobic bacteria [77].

2.10 Gallbladder motility

Defective gallbladder motility is another risk factor for cholesterol stones [78]. About one-third of patients with cholesterol gallstones display enlarged fasting and post prandial residual gallbladder volume with delayed emptying which antedates gallstone formation [79]. Sufficient time for cholesterol nucleation and gallstone growth is provided by dysfunctional gallbladder motility [80]. Various conditions are associated with dysfunctional gallbladder motility like insulin resistance, diabetes, irritable bowel syndrome, liver cirrhosis, and so on [81]. There is increase in lithogenic bile secretion to small intestine directly from liver in fasting motility defect, leading to faster recycling of bile acids and increasing bile acid pool hydrophobicity [82]. This is another predisposing factor for cholesterol crystallization and cholelithiasis [83].

3. Pathogenesis of gallstones

3.1 Cholesterol gallstones

Various defects occur simultaneously for the nucleation and crystallization of cholesterol monohydrate viz unphysiological supersaturation with cholesterol, accelerated nucleation and gallbladder hypomotility [16]. The mucin glycoprotein hypersecretion follows and lead to the stone formation [84].

Excessive secretion of cholesterol into bile leads to cholesterol supersaturation [85] owing to multiple biochemical defects either from increased input (de novo synthesis, lipoprotein uptake) or decreased disposition (de novo bile salt and cholesteryl ester synthesis) [84]. However single defects in hepatocellular processing of cholesterol are known viz

1. Increased number of apolipoprotein B/E and E receptors (constitutional/oestrogens/rapid weight loss/diet)

2. Increased activity of hydroxy-methyl-glutaryl-CoA reductase (obesity/hypertriglyceridemia/fibric acids)

3. Diminished activity of cholesterol 7α-hydroxylase (constitutional/fibric acids)

4. Diminished activity of Acyl CoA: cholesterol acyltransferase (constitutional/progestogens) [86]

These changes resulting in the increased levels of cholesterol in microsomes [87] and cytosol [88] of hepatocytes in patients with gallstones. Sterol carrier protein 2 concentration also increases simultaneously [89].

At puberty hypersecretion of cholesterol into bile begins [90]. In liver excess cholesterol is delivered to bile by a relay station [91]. Postprandially the cholesterol is completely micellized by bile salts and lecithin during healthy condition [92].

Cholesterol molecules are absorbed by gallbladder mucosa efficiently from micelles of supersaturated bile [93] where the activity of acyl coenzyme A: cholesterol acyl transferase esterifies the sterol [87]. But the molecules that remain free are dissolved in plasma and intercellular membranes where they become intercalated with and stiffen the phospholipid molecules [86]. Reverse diffusion when gallbladder bile become unsaturated or esterification is the only means of escape of membrane cholesterol as gallbladder mucosa does not produce cholesterol [92].

The abnormity in diurnal variation of gallbladder bile due to hypersecretion of cholesterol lead to the further trapping of excess free cholesterol molecules into gallbladder mucosa and muscle membranes [94]. There occurs the divergence of hepatic bile into gastrointestinal tract due to impaired motor and mucosal functions of gallbladder [95]. This in turn lead to increased bacterial catabolism and turnover of primary bile salts [92], which ultimately increase the production of secondary bile salts (hydrophobic bile salts) and suppress de novo bile salt synthesis [96].

Rapid recirculation and hydrophobicity are harmful for the stability of bile as these lead to the augmentation of secretion of cholesterol and hydrophobic lecithin molecules, which in turn shorten the time of nucleation of supersaturated bile [91]. The hydrophobicity of bile salt pool also increases secretion of total proteins into bile [97] and also altering the ratio of pro and anti-nucleating activities for cholesterol crystallization [97]. Multiple stimuli trigger mucin glycoprotein hypersecretion like cholesterol in itself [87], 'cytotoxic' filamentous cholesterol crystals [98], prostanoids [99], and hydrophobic bile salts e. g Deoxycholate and lithocholate conjugates [100]. This lead to the development of mucin gel on gallbladder wall and then as a crescent in gallbladder lumen, setting stage for accelerated nucleation. This together with hypomotility lead to its accumulation as biliary sludge, failure of complete evacuation of which lead to gallstone formation [84]. However, the end result may become inevitable by an environmental perturbation that inauspiciously tips the delicate pathophysiological and physical-chemical balance of supersaturated bile towards nucleation and stone growth [86].

3.2 Pigment gallstones

Black stones occur in sterile environment [101] with increased frequency in patients of chronic haemolysis. A shift in ratio of bilirubin diconjugates to the favour of monoconjugates especially monoglucuronides occur due to hypersecretion of bilirubin conjugates in bile [102]. Bile pigment output increases by 10-fold with haemolysis [102] and predominantly becomes monoconjugates that are more hydrolysed by endogenous β glucuronidase [101]. This gives rise to very high levels of unconjugated pigment exceeding biliary solubility [101]. The insoluble acid calcium salt [$Ca(HUCB)_2$] forms at pH values typical of gallbladder bile [103]. Unphysiological supersaturation occurs with an elevation in the ion product of calcium and monoacid species of unconjugated bilirubin [101] facilitating factors like in cholesterol stones are important for stone formation. The prevalence of pigment stones increases with age and is gender dependent; and all haemolytic patients does not develop pigment stones [101]. In experimental studies it was shown that there is no gallbladder motility defect in black pigment stone formation [104]. However, mucin hypersecretion occurs [105] in response to the high levels of unconjugated bilirubin [106] or mucosal cell cytotoxicity of earliest precipitates [107]. Nucleation is initiated at glandular crypts of gallbladder mucosa where mucin gel accumulates first [107]. Biliary supersaturation (owing to defective acidification of hepatic bile [101] with organic salts occur which is indicated by presence of crystalline calcium carbonate and phosphates in black pigment stones [101]. 3–20% of black pigment stones are composed of mucin glycoprotein [108]. Various factors came into play and through different mechanisms give rise to pigment stone formation in alcoholic cirrhosis, ileal dysfunction and in aging Viz bile salt hyposecretion, defective solubilization of unconjugated bilirubin, impaired calcium ion binding, haemolysis, defective bilirubin conjugation [101], enteric hyperbilirubinobilia [86].

Chronic anaerobic infection with functional stasis of bile ducts is necessary for brown pigment stones. Stasis in bile duct occur due to secondary stones from gallbladder, or due to sphincter of Oddi dysfunction or parasitic infections (mostly underdeveloped countries) [84]. Commencing with stasis of bile and then followed by anaerobic bacterial infection lead to accumulation of both mucin gel and bacterial cytoskeleton in bile ducts. Bacterial enzymes (phospholipase A, β glucuronidase) hydrolyse the biliary lipids that contain amide or ester linkages which results in the nucleation of cholesterol monohydrate crystals A trap is laid down in the form of culture medium for anaerobic bacteria by mucin gel and solid components making their exit difficult. This is a vicious cycle formed between growing stone, stasis of bile and bacterial infection [84, 109].

Author details

Mela Ram Attri[1], Irshad Ahmad Kumar[2]*, Ferkhand Mohi Ud Din[1], Ashiq Hussain Raina[1] and Aakarshit Attri[3]

1 Department of Surgery, Government Medical College, Srinagar, J&K, India

2 Directorate Health Services Kashmir, J&K, India

3 Government Medical College, Jammu, J&K, India

*Address all correspondence to: irshadahmadkumar@gmail.com

References

[1] Available from: https://www.niddk.nih.gov/health-information/digestive-diseases/gallstones

[2] Figueiredo J, Haiman C, Porcel J, et al. Sex and ethnic/racialspecific risk factors for gallbladder disease. BMC Gastroenterology. 2017;**17**(1):153

[3] Gupta SK, Shukla VK. Silent gallstones: A therapeutic dilemma (review). Tropical Gastroenterology. 2004;**25**:65-68

[4] Sanders G, Kingsnorth AN. Gallstones. British Medical Journal. 2007;**335**:295-299

[5] Schernhammer ES, Leitzmann MF, Michaud DS, Speizer FE, Giovannucci E, Colditz GA, et al. Cholecystectomy and the risk for developing colorectal cancer and distal colorectal adenomas. British Journal of Cancer. 2003;**88**:79-83

[6] Siddiqui AA, Kedika R, Mahgoub A, Patel M, Cipher DJ, Bapat V. A previous cholecystectomy increases the risk of developing advanced adenomas of the colon. Southern Medical Journal. 2009;**102**(11):1111-1115

[7] Huang D et al. Gallstones, cholecystectomy and the risk of hepatobiliary and pancreatic cancer: A nationwide population-based cohort study in Korea. Journal of Cancer Prevention. 2020;**25**(3):164-172. DOI: 10.15430/JCP.2020.25.3.164

[8] Hundal R, Shaffer EA. Gallbladder cancer: Epidemiology and outcome. Clinical Epidemiology. 2014;**6**:99-109

[9] Levy AD, Murakata LA, Rohrmann CA. Gallbladder carcinoma: Radiologic-pathologic correlation. Radiographics. 2001;**21**(2):295-314

[10] Ruhl CE, Everhart JE. Gallstone disease is associated with increased mortality in the United States. Gastroenterology. 2011;**140**(2):508-516

[11] Halldestam I, Enell EI, Kullman E, Borch K. Development of symptoms and complications in individuals with asymptomatic gallstones. British Journal of Surgery. 2004;**91**:734-738

[12] Tanaja J, Lopez RA, Meer JM. Cholelithiasis. StatPearls Publishing LLC. Available from: https://www.ncbi.nlm.nih.gov/books/NBK470440/

[13] Sandler RS, Everhart JE, Donowitz M, Adams E, Cronin K, Goodman C, et al. The burden of selected digestive disease in the United States. Gastroenterology. 2002;**122**:1500-1511

[14] Pak M, Lindseth G. Risk factors for cholelithiasis. Society of Gastroenterology Nurses and Associates. 2016;**39**(4). DOI: 10.1097/SGA.0000000000000235

[15] Apstein MD, Carey MC. Biliary tract stones and associated diseases. In: Stein JH, editor. Internal Medicine. 4th ed. St. Louis: Mosby Yearbook; 1993. [In press]

[16] Carey MC. Formation of cholesterol gallstones: The new paradigms. In: Paumgartner G, Stiehl A, Gerok W, editors. Trends in Bile Acid Research. Dordrecht: Kluwer; 1988. pp. 259-281

[17] Littlefield A, Lenahan C. Cholelithiasis: Presentation and Management. 1526-9523/09/$36.00. American College of Nurse-Midwives; 2019. DOI: 10.1111/jmwh.12959

[18] Sherlock S. Diseases of the Liver and Biliary System. 3rd ed. Oxford: Blackwell Scientific Publications; 1963

[19] Carey MC, Paigen B. Epidemiology of American Indian's burden and its

likely genetic origin. Hepatology. 2002;**36**:781-791

[20] Di Ciaula A, Wang DQH, Wang HH, Leonilde B, Portincasa P. Targets for current pharmacological therapy in cholesterol gallstone disease. Gastroenterology Clinics of North America. 2010;**39**:245-264. DOI: 10.1016/j.gtc2010.02.005

[21] Atamanalp SS, Keles MS, Atamanalp RS, Acemoglu H, Laloglu E. The effect of serum cholesterol, LDL, and HDL levels on gallstone cholesterol concentration. Pakistan Journal of Medical Science. 2013;**29**(1):187-190

[22] Kern F Jr. Effects of dietary cholesterol on cholesterol and bile acids homeostasis in patients with cholesterol gallstones. Journal of Clinical Investigation. 1994;**93**:1186-1194

[23] Portincasa P, Di Ciaula A, Wang HH, et al. Coordinate regulation of gallbladder motor function in the gut-liver axis. Hepatology. 2008;**47**: 2112-2126

[24] Volzke H, Baumeister SE, Alte D, Hoffmann W, Schwahn C, Simon P, et al. Independent risk factors for gallstone formation in a region with high cholelithaisis prevalence. Digestion. 2005;**71**:97-105

[25] Lammert F, Carey MC, Paigen B. Chromosomal organization of candidate genes involved in cholesterol gallstone formation: A murine gallstone map. Gastroenterology. 2001;**120**:221-238

[26] Jiang ZY, Parini P, Eggertsen G, et al. Increased expression of LXR alpha, ABCG5, ABCG8, and SR-BI in the liver from normolipidemic, nonobese Chinese gallstone patients. Journal of Lipid Research. 2008;**49**:464-472

[27] Hirobe-Jahn S, Harsch S, Renner O, et al. Association of FXR gene variants with cholelithiasis. Clinics and Research in Hepatology and Gastroenterology. 2015;**39**:68-79

[28] Martinez-Lopez E, Curiel-Lopez F, Hernandez-Nazara A, et al. Influence of ApoE and FABP2 polymorphisms and environmental factors in the susceptibility to gallstone disease. Annals of Hepatology. 2015;**14**: 515-523

[29] Chuang SC, Hsi E, Lee KT. Mucin genes in gallstone disease. Clinica Chimica Acta. 2012;**413**:1466-1471

[30] Chen Q, Li WJ, Wan YY, et al. Fibroblast growth factor receptor 4 Gly388Arg polymorphism associated with severity of gallstone disease in a Chinese population. Genetics and Molecular Research. 2012;**11**:548-555

[31] Miyasaka K, Takata Y, Funakoshi A. Association of cholecystokinin A receptor gene polymorphism with cholelithiasis and the molecular mechanisms of this polymorphism. Journal of Gastroenterology. 2002;**37**(Suppl 14):102-106

[32] Nakeeb A, Comuzzie AG, Martin L, et al. Gallstones: Genetics versus environment. Annals of Surgery. 2002;**235**:842-849

[33] Lammert F, Acalovschi M, Ercolani G, et al. EASL clinical practice guidelines on the prevention, diagnosis and treatment of gallstones. Journal of Hepatology. 2016;**65**:146-181

[34] Di Ciaula A, Portincasa P. Fat, epigenome and pancreatic diseases. Interplay and common pathways from a toxic and obesogenic environment. European Journal of Internal Medicine. 2014;**25**:865-873

[35] Moore KJ, Rayner KJ, Suarez Y, Fernandez-Hernando C. microRNAs and cholesterol metabolism. Trends in Endocrinology and Metabolism. 2010;**21**:699-706

[36] Yang B, Liu B, Bi P, et al. An integrated analysis of differential miRNA and mRNA expressions in human gallstones. Molecular BioSystems. 2015;**11**:1004-1011

[37] Wang R, Hong J, Cao Y, et al. Elevated circulating microRNA-122 is associated with obesity and insulin resistance in young adults. European Journal of Endocrinology. 2015;**172**:291-300

[38] Cirillo DJ, Wallace RB, Rodabough RJ, Greenland P, LaCroix AZ, Limacher MC, et al. Effect of estrogen therapy on gallbladder disease. JAMA: The Journal of the American Medical Association. 2005;**293**(3):330-339

[39] Moghaddam TG, Fakheri H, Abdi R, Rostami FK, Bari Z. The incidence and outcome of pregnancy-related biliary sludge/stones and potential risk factors. Achieves of Iranian Medicine. 2013;**16**(10):12-16

[40] Racine A, Bijon A, Fournier A, Mesrine S, Clavel-Chapelon F, Carbonnel F, et al. Menopausal hormone therapy and risk of cholecystectomy: A prospective study based on the French E3N cohort. Canadian Medical Association Journal. 2013;**185**(7):555-561

[41] Everhart JE, Yeh F, Lee ET, Hill MC, Fabsitz R, Howard BV, et al. Prevalence of gallbladder disease in American Indian populations: Findings from the strong heart study. Hepatology. 2002;**35**(6):1507-1512

[42] Dutta U, Nagi B, Garg PK, Sinha SK, Singh K, Tandon RK. Patients with gallstones develop gallbladder cancer at an earlier age. European Journal of Cancer Prevention. 2005;**14**:381-385

[43] Grimaldi CH, Nelson RG, Pettitt DJ, Sampliner RE, Bennett PH, Knowler WC. Increased mortality with gallstone disease: Results of a 20-year population-based survey in Pima Indians. Annals of Internal Medicine. 1993;**118**(3):185-190

[44] Han TQ, Jiang ZY, Suo GJ, Zhang SD. Apolipoprotein B-100 gene Xba 1 polymorphism and cholesterol gallstone disease. Clinical Genetics. 2000;**57**(4):304-308

[45] Venneman NG, Van Erpecum KJ. Pathogenesis of gallstones. Gastroenterology Clinics of North America. 2010;**39**(2):171-183

[46] Andreotti G, Chen J, Gao YT, Rashid A, Chang SC, Shen MC, et al. Serum lipid levels and the risk of biliary stones: A population-based study in China. International Journal of Cancer. 2008;**122**(10):2322-2329

[47] Acalovschi M. Cholesterol gallstones: From epidemiology to prevention. Postgraduate Medical Journal. 2001;**77**:221-229

[48] Tsai CJ, Leitzmann MF, Willett WC, Giovannucci EL. Glycemic load, glycemic index, and carbohydrate intake in relation to risk of cholecystectomy in women. Gastroenterology. 2005;**129**: 105-112

[49] Biddinger SB, Haas JT, Yu BB, Bezy O, Jing E, Zhang W, et al. Hepatic insulin resistance directly promotes formation of cholesterol gallstones. Nature Medicine. 2008;**14**:778-782

[50] Shaffer EA, Small DM. Biliary lipid secretion in cholesterol gallstone disease: The effect of cholecystectomy and obesity. Journal of Clinical Investigation. 1977;**59**:828-840

[51] Tsai CJ, Leitzmann MF, Hu FB, Willett WC, Giovannucci EL. A prospective cohort study of nut consumption and the risk of gallstone disease. American Journal of Epidemiology. 2004;**160**(1):961-968

[52] Leitzmann MF, Stampfer MJ, Willett WC, Spiegelman D, Colditz GA, Giovannucci EL. Coffee intake is associated with lower risk of symptomatic gallstone disease in women. Gastroenterology. 2002;**123**:1823-1830

[53] Misciagna G, Centonze S, Leoci C, Guerra V, Cisternino AM, Ceo R, et al. Diet, physical activity, and gallstones: A population-based, case-control study in Southern Italy. American Journal of Clinical Nutrition. 1999;**69**:120-126

[54] Mendez-Sanchez N, Gonzalez V, Aguayo P, Sanchez JM, Tanimoto MA, Elizondo J, et al. Fish oil (n-3) polyunsaturated fatty acids beneficially affect biliary cholesterol nucleation time in obese women losing weight. Journal of Nutrition. 2001;**131**(9):2300-2303

[55] Moerman CJ, Smeets FW, Kromhout D. Dietary risk factors for clinically diagnosed gallstones in middle-aged men. A 25 year follow-up study (the Zutphen study). Annuals of Epidemiology. 1994;**4**:248-254

[56] Simon JA, Hudes ES. Serum ascorbic acid and gallbladder disease prevalence among US adults: The Third National Health and Nutrition Examination Survey. JAMA: The Journal of the American Medical Association, Internal Medicine. 2000;**160**:931-936

[57] Tsai CJ, Leitzmann MF, Willett WC, Giovannucci EL. Fruit and vegetable consumption and risk of cholecystectomy in women. American Journal of Medicine. 2006;**119**:760-767

[58] Stampfer MJ, Maclure KM, Colditz GA, Manson JE, Willett WC. Risk of symptomatic gallstones in women with severe obesity. American Journal of Clinical Nutrition. 1992;**55**(3):652-658

[59] Li VK, Pulido N, Fajnwaks P, Szomstein S, Rosenthal R, Martinez-Duartez P. Predictors of gallstone formation after bariatric surgery: A multivariate analysis of risk factors comparing gastric bypass, gastric banding, and sleeve gastrectomy. Surgical Endoscopy. 2009;**23**:1640-1644

[60] Leitzmann MF, Rimm EB, Willett WC, Splegelman D, Grodstein F, Stampfer MJ, et al. Recreational physical activity and the risk of cholecystectomy in women. The New England Journal of Medicine. 1999;**341**(11):777-784

[61] Watkins JB, Crawford ST, Sanders RA. Chronic voluntary exercise may alter hepatobiliary clearance of endogenous and exogenous chemicals in rats. Drug Metabolism and Disposition. 1994;**22**:537-543

[62] Dubrac S, Parquet M, Blouquit Y, Gripois D, Blouquit MF, Souidi M, et al. Insulin injections enhance cholesterol gallstone incidence by changing the biliary cholesterol saturation index and apo A-1 concentration in hamsters fed a lithogenic diet. Journal of Hepatology. 2001;**35**:550-557

[63] Kirwan JP, Kohrt WM, Wojta DW, Bourey RE, Holloszy JO. Endurance exercise training reduces glucose-stimulated insulin levels in 60- to 70-year-old men and women. Journal of Gerontology. 1993;**48**:M84-M90

[64] Leitzmann MF, Giovannucci EL, Rimm EB, Stampfer MJ, Spiegelman D, Wing AL, et al. The relation of physical activity to risk for symptomatic gallstone disease in men. Annual Internal Medicine. 1998;**128**:417-425

[65] Buzas C, Chira O, Mocan T, Acalovschi M. Comparative study of gallbladder mortality in patients with chronic HCV hepatitis and with HCV cirrhosis. Romanian Journal of Internal Medicine. 2011;**49**(1):37-44

[66] Acalovschi M, Buzas C, Grigorescu M. Hepatitis C virus

infection is a risk factor for gallstone disease: A prospective hospital-based study of patients with chronic viral C hepatitis. Journal of Viral Hepatology. 2009;**16**:860-866

[67] Al-Azzawi HH, Mathur A, Lu D, Swartz-Basile DA, Nakeeb A, Pitt HA. Resistin-like molecule α reduces gallbladder optima tension. Journal of Gastrointestinal Surgery. 2007;**11**:95-100

[68] Ruhl CE, Everhart JE. Association of diabetes, serum insulin, and C-peptide with gallbladder disease. Hepatology. 2000;**31**:299-303

[69] Ahmed MH, Barakat S, Almobarak AO. The association between renal stone disease and cholesterol gallstones: The easy to believe and not hard to retrieve theory of the metabolic syndrome. Renal Failure. 2014;**36**(6):957-962

[70] Stinton LM, Myers RP, Shaffer EA. Epidemiology of gallstones. Gastroenterology Clinics of North America. 2010;**39**:157-169

[71] Sahi T, Paffenbarger RS, Hsieh CC, Lee IM. Body mass index, cigarette smoking, and other characteristics as predictors predictors of self-reported, physician-diagnosed gallbladder disease in male college alumni. American Journal of Epidemiology. 1998;**147**:644-651

[72] Murray FE, Logan RF, Hannaford PC, Kay CR. Cigarette smoking and parity as risk factors for the development of symptomatic gall bladder disease in women: Results of the Royal College of General Practitioners' Oral contraception study. Gut. 1994;**35**:107-111

[73] Walcher T, Haenle M, Mason RA, Konig W, Imhof A, Kratzer W. The effect of alcohol, tobacco, and caffeine consumption and vegetarian diet on gallstone prevalence. European Journal of Gastroenterology and Hepatology. 2010;**22**:1345-1351

[74] Wang DQ, Zhang L, Wang HH. High cholesterol absorption efficiency and rapid biliary secretion of chylomicron remnant cholesterol enhance cholelithogenesis in gallstone-susceptible mice. Biochimica et Biophysica Acta. 2005;**1733**:90-99

[75] Wang DQ. Regulation of intestinal cholesterol absorption. Annual Review of Physiology. 2007;**69**:221-248

[76] Wu T, Zhang Z, Liu B, et al. Gut microbiota dysbiosis and bacterial community assembly associated with cholesterol gallstones in large-scale study. BMC Genomics. 2013;**14**:669

[77] Thomas LA, Veysey MJ, Murphy GM, et al. Octreotide induced prolongation of colonic transit increases faecal anaerobic bacteria, bile acid metabolising enzymes, and serum deoxycholic acid in patients with acromegaly. Gut. 2005;**54**:630-635

[78] Portincasa P, Moschetta A, Palasciano G. Cholesterol gallstone disease. Lancet. 2006;**368**:230-239

[79] Portincasa P, Di Ciaula A, Baldassarre G, et al. Gallbladder motor function in gallstone patients: Sonographic and in vitro studies on the role of gallstones, smooth muscle function and gallbladder wall inflammation. Journal of Hepatology. 1994;**21**:430-440

[80] Portincasa P, Di Ciaula A, vanBerge-Henegouwen GP. Smooth muscle function and dysfunction in gallbladder disease. Current Gastroenterology Reports. 2004;**6**:151-162

[81] Ciaula AD, Wang DQ-H, Portincas P. An Update on the Pathogenesis of Cholesterol Gallstone

Disease. Wolters Kluwer Health, Inc.; DOI:10.1097/MOG.0000000000000423

[82] vanBerge-Henegouwen GP, Venneman NG, Portincasa P, et al. Relevance of hereditary defects in lipid transport proteins for the pathogenesis of cholesterol gallstone disease. Scandinavian Journal of Gastroenterology. Supplement. 2004:60-69

[83] van Erpecum KJ, Portincasa P, Gadellaa M, et al. Effects of bile salt hydrophobicity on nucleation behaviour of cholesterol crystals in model bile. European Journal of Clinical Investigation. 1996;**26**:602-608

[84] Reshetnyak VI. Concept of the pathogenesis and treatment of cholelithiasis. World Journal of Hepatology. 2012;**4**(2):18-34. DOI: 10.4254/wjh.v4.i2.18

[85] Hofmann AF. Bile acid secretion, bile flow and biliary lipid secretion in humans. Hepatology. 1990;**12**:17S-25S

[86] LaMont JT, Carey MC. Cholesterol gallstone formation. 2. Pathobiology and pathomechanics. Progress in Liver Diseases. 1992;**10**:165-191

[87] Sahlin S, Ablberg J, Reihnrr E, S~thlberg D, Einarsson K. Cholesterol metabolism in human gallbladder mucosa: Relationship to cholesterol gallstone disease and effects of chenodeoxycholic acid and ursodeoxycholic acid treatment. Hepatology. 1992;**16**:320-326

[88] Smith JL, Hardic IR, Pillay SP, de Jersey J. Hepatic acylcoenzyme A: Cholesterol acyltransferase activity is decreased in patients with cholesterol gallstones. Journal of Lipid Research. 1990;**31**:1993-2000

[89] Kawata S, Imai Y, Inada M, et al. Modulation of cholesterol 7a-hydroxylase activity by non-specific lipid transfer protein in human liver--possibly altered regulation of its cytosolic level in patients with gallstones. Clinica Chimica Acta. 1991;**197**:201-208

[90] Von Bergmann K, Becker M, Leiss O. Biliary cholesterol saturation in non-obese women and non-obese men before and after puberty. European Journal of Clinical Investigation. 1986;**16**:531-535

[91] Carey MC, LaMont JT. Cholesterol gallstone formation. 1. Physical-chemistry of bile and biliary lipid secretion. Progress in Liver Diseases. 1992;**10**:139-163

[92] Carey MC, Cahalane MJ. Enterohepatic circu!ation. In: Arias IM, Jacoby WB, Popper H, Schacter D, Shafritz D, editors. The Liver: Biology and Pathobiology. New York: Raven Press; 1988. pp. 573-616

[93] Carey MC, Hernell O. Fat digestion and absorption. Seminars in Gastrointestinal Disease. 1992;**3**:189-208

[94] Metzger AL, Adler R, Heymsfield S, Grundy SM. Diurnal variation in biliary lipid composition. The New England Journal of Medicine. 1973;**288**:333-336

[95] Roslyn JJ, DenBesten L, Thompson JE, Cohen K. Chronic cholelithiasis and decreased bile salt pool size: Cause or effect? American Journal of Surgery. 1980;**139**:119-124

[96] Vlahcevic ZR, Heuman DM, Hylemon PB. Regulation of bile acid synthesis. Hepatology. 1991;**13**:590-600

[97] Jiingst D, Lang T, Ritter C, Paumgartner G. Role of high total protein in gallbladder bile in the formation of cholesterol gallstones. Gastroenterology. 1991;**100**:1724-1729

[98] Konikoff FM, Chung DS, Donovan JM, Small DM, Carey MC.

Filamentous, helical and tubular microstructures during cholesterol crystallization from bile. Evidence that biliary cholesterol does not nucleate classic monohydrate plates. The Journal of Clinical Investigation. 1992;**90**: 1156-1161

[99] Carey MC, Cahalane MJ. Whither biliary sludge? Gastroenterology. 1988;**95**:508-523

[100] Carey MC. Physical-chemical properties of bile acids and their salts. In: Danielsson H, Sjrvall H, editors. Sterols and Bile Acids. Amsterdam: Elsevier; 1985. pp. 345-403

[101] Cahalane MJ, Neubrand MW, Carey MC. Physical-chemical pathogenesis of pigment gallstones. Seminars in Liver Disease. 1988;**8**: 317-328

[102] Fevery J, Blanckaert NB, Leroy P, Michiels R, Heirwegh KPM. Analysis of bilirubins in biological fluids by extraction and thin-layer chromatography of the intact tetrapyrrols: Application to bile of patients with Gilbert's syndrome, hemolysis or cholelithiasis. Hepatology. 1983;**3**:177-183

[103] Ostrow JD. Unconjugated bilirubin and cholesterol gallstone formation. Hepatology. 1990;**12**:219S-226S

[104] Behar J, Lee KY, Thompson WR, Brancani P. Gallbladder contraction in patients with pigment and cholesterol stones. Gastroenterology. 1989;**97**: 1479-1484

[105] Malet PF, Deng S-Q, Soloway RD. Gallbladder mucin and cholesterol and pigment gallstone formation in hamsters. Scandinavian Journal of Gastroenterology. 1984;**24**:1055-1060

[106] Trotman BW, Bernstein SE, Balistreri WF, Wirt GD, Martin RA. Hemolysis induced gallstones in mice: Increased unconjugated bilirubin in hepatic bile predisposes to gallstone formation. Gastroenterology. 1981;**81**:232-236

[107] Trotman BD, Bongiovanni MB, Kahn MJ, Bernstein SE. A morphological study of the liver and gallbladder in hemolysis-induced gallstone disease in mice. Hepatology. 1982;**2**:863-869

[108] Carey MC. Pathogenesis of gallstones. Recenti Progressi in Medicina. 1992;**83**:379-391

[109] Uchiyama K, Kawai M, Tani M, Terasawa H, Tanimura H, Yamaue H. Pathogenesis of hepatolithiasis based on the analysis of components of intrahepatic stones. Hepato-Gastroenterology. 2007;**54**:1798-1804